This book is dedicated to my husband, Michael Gordon. I will never be able to thank him for everything he has done for me and our children. The sacrifices he's made, the unconditional love and compassion that he would shower us with every day, his unwavering loyalty to our family, the vision for the future, the kind way he would make us feel that everything would be okay, the strength that he portrayed that made him bigger than life to everyone that he met, his dedication to work to provide well for his family, his sense of humor which he would use to lighten up anyone's day who crossed paths with him, the way he would forgive without question, and hug and kiss everyone telling them constantly how much he loved them every day. Yes God blessed me with the most incredible husband and best friend in the whole universe. Knowing him has been a privilege. Sharing our life together has been a blessing and I love him more than I could ever express in words or deeds. He is always going to be "The Absolute Love of My Life!"

Thank You to All our Family and Friends

I would like to Thank God absolutely first for all his blessings. I want to thank Joel Olsteen and his ministries for all his positive messages and motivational services that have helped motivate and keep us believing that God has Michael in the palm of his hand. I want to thank all our family, friends, and church family that have gone out of their way in many ways throughout this journey. Many of you helped us financially, emotionally, physically and spiritually. Thank you to all those people and many that we don't even know who have prayed for us in their churches, their homes and other venues. The power of prayer is alive and well. May God Bless each and every one of you!

Contents

Chapter One

This book is about the journey that my husband, Michael and I have been going through since August 2013. It is important to give a picture of what our life and dreams were at that time and how life can change in an instant.

Michael had just reached a point in his life where he wanted to work on his passion which was prospecting. He had invented many things over the years but as most of us can do, he got side tracked and never completed the process. Michael had invented a gold processing machine that he had designed years previously and was hopeful to put it in production on a working gold mining claim. He had offers from all over the world from Mali, Columbia and the United States but it seemed that eventually they would all fall through. He was an expert in the process of finding and production of gold, and performing these tasks in an affordable way. Because of his expertise, knowledge about gold production and the price of gold rising as it was, Michaels' opinion and expertise was in high demand. The professionals and investors who were used to dealing in oil production, coal mining, and other types of investments were not real familiar or comfortable with gold mining. The last thing they wanted was to get ripped off or invest in a bad claim. Many of these guys would email project after project asking for Michaels' opinion of the project. At times it was frustrating because Michael spent hours working to help these guys and would never receive any compensation. Michael would tell me it will work out in the end. He believed that eventually he would find the right project and he would be rewarded for all his hard work and knowledge.

Michael's dream was to be in the Arizona desert and enjoying the world of prospecting. I was excited for him to achieve it. He had always put our family first and done whatever was required to meet our family's wants and needs throughout the years. He loved us all unconditionally, the children, the grandchildren and I can testify emphatically to that. With the children grown and married, it was now his time to do what he loved and desired, to be a prospector.

His goal wasn't just to be a full time prospector or an operator of a gold claim but to be in the environment that he really enjoys and loves. Michael had been prospecting since he was little in Oregon and again in his twenties in Idaho when he was working for the Forest Service. At that time he had designed a machine to use to help him find more gold faster than by hand panning. Although it was small it was perfect for him at that time. Throughout the years I heard all about it and how he wanted to manufacture these machines and how great they would be for numerous miners. He especially thought they would make a fantastic fit for people in third world countries that had no electricity or fuel for other types of machines. His vision was to help others and of course help us financially at the same time. He has a heart of "gold" you could say.

During several years previous to August, 2013 many different projects were emailed to him for his professional opinion to see if they were a viable project and worthy of an investors time. Most of them would receive his thumb down. But one really got his attention. It was in Arizona and he believed it meant "big gold." Michael and our son-in-law drove out there to look at the project personally to see if it truly was a good project. Michael performed some test samples himself to see the potential of the property. He took our machine with him so he could use it for the tests. The trip proved very positive. He was impressed with the owner but most of all with the property. There were hard rock mines and placer claims and the owner had the property on the market to sell. It was the richest claim he had ever seen.

The owner spent the next several years learning from Michael and using his expertise to help him in the effort to sell the hard rock mines and placer claims as a package deal together or separate. Over the next several years Michael went out to Arizona to take samples, he documented his findings, performed the concentrating of the material, and sent the concentrate to a lab for updated results for potential buyers. He met several different interested parties at the property for the owner so he could answer any questions about the property or in case the potential buyer would like to talk to Michael about being the operator to produce the property after they purchased it.

Even though there seemed to be setback after setback Michael remained steadfast. He really believed in this project and through it all was looking forward to getting into the Arizona sun and desert spending time prospecting or producing this property.

In August 2013, Michael was contacted by another group of owners who wanted him to help them design a platform that they could use on their project in another city in Arizona. The main problem most owners had that wanted to put their properties into production was the desert did not have easy access to water or electricity. Michael had solved that problem with a design he had come up with that included a self contained water source that would re-circulate and that also had a solar power source for continued power for production. The gold recovery machine he had invented was not part of this platform he would design for these claim owners. He did use the solar and re-circulating system on this property. Each property can have a different set of challenges but most would have the water, electricity or power problem. This property had several other challenges with magnetite so Michael worked on a design for a platform that would lift the magnetite from the material as it went through the platform. He was a wonderful trouble shooter and could find an answer pretty quick in any endeavor he undertook. That is why people wanted him on site whether we were building something in construction or these platforms. This particular design he would name the "Blue Rose".

He was excited about getting out there in Arizona and helping these guys put together the platform they could use for their specific needs. It was during this time frame Michael had been having trouble with food feeling like it was getting stuck in his esophagus when he would swallow. I insisted he see a doctor and one evening in August 2013 we went to a Hospital Emergency Room in Tulsa, Oklahoma. He described his symptoms and we were hopeful they could help him feel better and fix this feeling he was having when he ate. The hospital took several tests and eventually they determined that Michael had acid reflux and maybe an ulcer and they wrote a prescription for him to take that was called "magic mouthwash".

We got the prescription filled and when he used the magic mouthwash it appeared to help by numbing his esophagus. Our son, Larry, had needed Michael's advice on a project he was doing and came over to pick him up and was shocked at how much weight Michael had lost. Our son started researching and talking to a natural health expert he knew. He called and told us that he was bringing over a liquid called "Samento" and some salt tablets. This was supposed to help what we thought Michael had been battling for several years, "Lyme Disease." It was Lyme disease that we originally thought was the reason he was losing so much weight. We believed this because a doctor several years earlier diagnosed him with Lyme and dispensed antibiotics to help it. For more medical history, Michael had also been in a severe wreck in 2005 and had suffered from a back injury that created much pain in his lower back and caused his nerves in his legs to constantly jump. One of his doctors performed several epidurals with no long term help. The eventual goal was back surgery but we were not in a hurry for that. Laser surgery was a possibility but affording that option was not a possibility at this time so that was put on hold. The doctor he went to for this wreck referred him to a pain management doctor because the pain he was experiencing was ongoing. The pain management doctor started scheduling Michael every month or so for a checkup and would be instrumental in helping him deal with the discomfort and pain that he lived with because of the wreck. The pain doctor would also continue to renew his magic mouthwash prescription as he needed it. This doctor knew Michael's medical history, the Lyme disease, the car wreck, and they also discussed the problems Michael had been having with his eating. The doctor told him that if it didn't get better soon he needed to see a GI doctor and that he could refer him to one he knew.

Michael appreciated this doctor's opinion but because Michael had been told he was suffering from acid reflux and thought he had the proper medicine to help with that diagnosis Michael went ahead and scheduled to go to Arizona and help those owners with their platform. He spent several months there and was successful in his effort to design a platform they could use for their specific property. During his time in Arizona he thought it might be fun for me to come out and spend a couple of days with him. I thought that was a fantastic idea and could not wait to go. I made arrangements for my flight and looked forward to spending some quality time with him.

He had planned a fantastic trip for me. It would be the absolute best time we have ever had. He picked me up from the airport and believe me we both had butterflies waiting to see the other. I was constantly watching my phone and could track where he was and where I was on an app I had on my phone. I loved how we slowly were moving closer and closer to each other.

As soon as he picked me up he wanted to show me where he had been staying in Arizona with one of the owners and his brother. They had rented a house in a retirement community. After that stop we went over to where the platform was that he was designing. He wanted me to meet the owner and his brother who were also at the platform and he wanted me to see what he had been creating. It was impressive and I was extremely proud of him. The owner and his brother kept telling me how knowledgeable Michael was and excited they all were to get the project going. They also knew Michael had been working long and hard on their project so they told us both it was great I had come to see him and that he was looking forward to spending several days visiting with me. So off we went on our next adventure.

We weren't far from the well known Superstition Mountains and he has been excited to take me there. He had spent some thought on what we could do during my visit. First we stopped at the Superstition Mountain Museum and it was interesting and informative. We both love the movie "Tombstone" so the next place on the itinerary was Tombstone, Arizona. We enjoyed the drive but most of all just being together was priceless. We spent hours talking about how wonderful our life was going to be in Arizona, our dreams, and all the fun we were going to have.

In Tombstone, Arizona we found a cute little old motel and believe me the feel was old, rustic with the appearance of the old days. As soon as we got unpacked we started walking around the town. The town was just as you would guess, old and rustic, wood floor plank walkways in front of all the shops just like in the movies. They had many planned events, including a performance of a shooting at the OK Corral. We took in as many events as we could and we enjoyed souvenir shopping but most of all we were enjoying each other and holding hands just like newlyweds. Although we were enjoying the feeling of the old west and visiting Tombstone, Michael said we were going to get a nicer room the next night when we went to Phoenix. He had planned on taking me to the Arizona State Fair and then he told me that Trace Adkins was performing at the fair. He said "why don't you see if you can get us tickets, I know you'd enjoy seeing Trace in concert." I was able to get a couple of tickets so the concert was added to the itinerary. We woke up in Tombstone the next day, packed and got on the road, destination Phoenix.

I was able to get a reservation close to the fair at a Best Western Inn. This motel room was fantastic. The room was called the "Cactus Wren suite". It had all the amenities that you would expect of a really nice hotel especially compared to the one the night before. As soon as we checked in we began unpacking and preparing for the concert and the fair. We both were on the top of the world. When we were ready to go to the fair, Michael had the front desk call a cab that they recommended. When the cab driver picked us up, Michael got his phone number and paid him well to come back and pick us up when we were done at the fair. We always enjoyed going to the fair and this one was in another city and a new adventure. It was time for the concert so we went there first. After the concert we rode the Ferris wheel. We always enjoyed that. It is always romantic and at night very beautiful with the lights and all the sites. We walked around the fair, got something to eat and drink and then we saw a place that made wood carvings. Michael wanted something special made and decided on a beautiful plaque that had 2 hearts together with Michael & Joyce burnt into the wood and a Blue Rose. I took a picture with him holding it. He looked so handsome, happy and his beautiful smile bright as the sun. We were so happy, excited about our future, looking forward to eventually moving to Arizona and living the dream. We had no idea that this trip would mean more than we could ever imagine. You never know what the future holds and I must confess this was the most wonderful trip but it would mean even more to us in a couple of months from then. The next morning was the day I was due to return to Tulsa, Oklahoma. He wanted to take me shopping in the mall, where he bought me an awesome watch and then we went to eat at PF Changs. This was somewhere he had been telling me he wanted to take me to while I was there. It was a great place to eat. We did not know at the time that this fantastic lunch would be one of our last meals out together. After lunch we took the slow drive to the airport and believe me we both dreaded it. We have always loved being together and although we knew we both had responsibilities we hated being apart. Michael talked the airport personnel into being able to walk me to my gate, and he sat and waited with me until I boarded. He carried my bag and reminded me how very much he loved me, although he has always showed me and told me that throughout every day in every way, this time he wanted me to know that being apart was temporary and kept reminding me to keep my mind on the prize the fantastic new chapter of our life in Arizona. I flew home and he went back to finish his work designing the platform for the claim owners in Arizona. Michael completed his agreement in Arizona in November 2013.

During this time he was also in contact with the owner of the property he called "big gold" and they both decided since Michael was out there maybe he should go by on his way back home and get some samples so he would have them in his possession should they need them later on. Michael was able to spend some quality time that he cherished walking throughout that property doing some sampling and picking up some awesome rocks to bring back home to me. Several rocks contained gold throughout. When he would call me he would be so excited and overwhelmed about how wonderful the property is for gold production. As Michael drove home to Oklahoma he would call and tell me that he was super excited about his trip, the samples he retrieved at the "big gold" and the general terrain of the area. All he would talk about was he could not wait to get back and prospect that property or sell it so we could get our very own property to prospect. He told me over and over I can't wait until we get back out there prospecting in the desert.

Chapter Two

While Michael was gone he had been using the magic mouthwash the hospital told him to take, the Samento and sometimes the salt tablets at times throughout the period between August 2013 and November 2013 while he was in Arizona. It had appeared to help but he still was eating less, smaller bites, and had been losing weight. Michael had been losing weight for a year but we thought that was because of the Lyme disease. Michael had weighed 280-300 pounds before and his height was 6 foot 6 inches. He preferred to be at about 240 pounds but now he was closer to 200 pounds.

It started to become harder and harder for Michael to swallow the medicines that he was on. One medicine in particular was Gabapentin. This medicine is a large tablet that would get stuck in his esophagus. It would take Michael rocking back and forth to get it to go on past his esophagus to his stomach.

Thanksgiving 2013 was a wonderful day with our family. Michael was sharing with everyone samples of rocks he had found at the "big gold" property on his way back from Arizona. He shared stories and everyone enjoyed listening to him, especially our grandkids.

Christmas 2013 came and although we had a wonderful day with our family, everyone could tell that Michael seemed to be losing more weight. It appeared Michael was having more and more trouble getting food and medicine to go through his esophagus. It became harder and more upsetting to him that he couldn't eat his food. I had mentioned to him several times that he should see a doctor but Michael was not really fond of doctors since he had spent many months in the hospital in Germany during his time in the Army because of a parachuting accident. This incident made him wary of going back to the hospital for anything. I understood but eventually I had to really insist that he needed to go in and get checked.

Finally on March 7, 2014, I convinced Michael that he needed to get checked out so late that evening we drove to a Hospital in downtown Tulsa, Oklahoma. I knew Michael was nervous and I was nervous as well but I was happy he was going in to get checked and I prayed that he could find out the problem and get well and we could go on down the road in our life, healthy and whole.

Describing the symptoms to the doctor, loss of weight, food getting stuck in his esophagus, and his medicine getting stuck, the doctor ordered several tests. Lab tests came back great. The doctor told us by the lab results he appears extremely healthy. The doctor ordered a series of tests that included x-rays, CAT scan with barium, and other tests. The doctor then told us that it appears he has a hiatal hernia. I was pleasantly happy about this; I knew that this is treatable. The doctor told us the test he really needed to have was an endoscope. The doctor told us that during that procedure it was a possibility that the doctor could stretch his esophagus and he would be able to eat better. We were told that a special GI doctor could perform the endoscope the next morning. This meant that Michael would need to stay in the hospital, so he could be prepped for the procedure in the morning. Although Michael was not happy about that scenario he agreed because he believed that if the doctor was successful he could eat a steak on the way home. He was then moved from the emergency room to a regular room on another floor in the hospital.

The room he was moved to was not a private room and there was another patient already in that room that was suffering from pneumonia.

This patient also had claustrophobia and would not allow the door to the room to be closed. Another patient down the hall kept whining and screaming constantly. It was a horrifying sound that made your skin crawl and was not what you wanted to hear when you weren't that comfortable in hospitals and were looking at going under anesthesia and possibly surgery the next morning. We complained and complained to the nurses but they said there was nothing that they could do. Michael looked at me in horror and I knew he hated being here but he would endure it so we could get this procedure done in an effort to get him healthy and also because he knew he really wanted to eat a steak.

He told me to go home and take care of our pets and try to get some rest so I could be there early in the morning. It was already 2 in the morning so I wasn't going to get much sleep but I did as he requested so I could take care of our pets. I figured that how it had been going in the hospital, Michael wasn't going to get much sleep either. I gave him a kiss, went home, and took care of our pets.

Instead of sleeping I got on my computer and started researching everything possible that had the same type of symptoms that he had. I have to admit I was scared to death, especially with the potential possibilities. I just kept hoping and waiting to find out what was causing the problems he was having and praying that it could be treated and fixed quickly and easily. I knew if he did have a hernia that would require surgery. Michael would dread surgery because his dad had died during an operation and he had mentioned dying in surgery numerous times. Even though I was aware of what the possibilities were, I just kept praying and believing for the best case scenario and praying that we would get good news in the morning.

March 9, 2014, was endoscopy procedure day. I went back to the hospital early so I could be there with him and give him support, love and encouragement before the procedure. I knew he did not like being in the hospital. I also knew he had to be nervous.

We spent numerous hours talking about how great it is going to be when the doctor performing the endoscope stretched his esophagus so he could eat much easier. This is the outcome we were both looking forward to. We discussed where we were going to go eat when he got out of the hospital. He told me we are going to Red Lobster, Olive Garden but most importantly he wanted steak. Then the nurse came to get him for the procedure, I kissed him, told him I loved him and off they went.

I went to wait as others do that accompany their loved ones during these types of procedures. Although I was extremely anxious waiting for the procedure to be over, the main thought going through my head was, just hurry up and please come tell me everything's ok and that the procedure went well.

It seemed like forever, but eventually I was called back into a room with a lazy boy chair and a couple of other chairs. I sat there for a few more minutes and then through the door the doctor walked in who had a name I could not pronounce. As he entered the room and without not even getting entirely in the room he immediately said to me, "It's really bad, very bad." I just looked at him in shock. What does that mean? I ask him, "What do you mean by that?" He started to tell me very unsympathetically and with a demeanor that shouted he could care less about Michael or me, he said "he has a tumor that he absolutely believes is cancer but the biopsy that he sent off for testing will prove it for sure. He waited too long to come in here." I said what can we do if he's having trouble eating? He said "Get a feeding tube. He just waited too long." I asked if Michael knew and he said no. And he left. I was in shock, heart broken, lost, scared, and didn't know which way to turn. I went out of the room, not knowing which way to go, what to do, I walked out the first door I saw, and it went out to a garage at the hospital. Before I got outside into the garage it hit me even more intensely what was unfolding in our life. I had just taken my phone and dialed my mom and when she answered; all I could do was start crying hysterically, (which is not like me). As I cried I started to tell her what had happened, and what the doctor said, and that Michael didn't know, and oh my God, mom what are we going to do! The more I told her the more visions came to me about what was happening, Michael has cancer, Michael may die, Oh my god, what are we going to do, we have no money, no insurance, Oh my god, what are we going to do, he doesn't know, how is he going to handle it, my heart just broke into pieces. I felt helpless. My mom asked me where are the kids? I didn't know so she tried to calm me down and said she would call them and get them down there. She didn't feel that I should be alone. I told her I need to meet Michael back in his room after he gets out of recovery.

In the meantime our daughter, Eden, called and said, "Mom, I will meet you at the front entrance, I am almost there." I went to the front entrance waiting for Eden as she requested, still crying, replaying what the doctor had said, scanning my brain that I can't believe this, this can't be real, it can't be happening to us, and what is Michael going to do when he finds out. Michael had spoken many times about if he got sick with something pretty devastating he wouldn't want to endure it. Especially if it caused him to be in a wheelchair, on life support or other debilitating illness. This played over in my mind with everything else and I just felt helpless and scared.

I saw Eden being dropped off in front of the hospital and she walked in and gave me a hug, immediately I started crying uncontrollably and it's like my legs were rubber bands because I had a hard time standing up. I was just so overwhelmed. Eden kept hugging me, trying to console me, and trying to give me what little words of encouragement she could muster as I knew she was devastated as well. She has just received the same news from her grandmother and on top of that here is her mother a total complete mess. I am sure she was overwhelmed with seeing me in the condition I was in as well. She helped me go to the floor Michael was being taken back to where his room was. One by one our oldest daughter, Christie, our son, Larry and our son-in-laws showed up in the waiting room to offer support. As we sat in the waiting room, I just kept crying and dreading when Michael got back to his room. How do you tell someone you love they have cancer? How can you do that? Eden went to ask for the doctor who had been treating him on the floor he was on, not the doctor who had performed his endoscope, but the doctor assigned to him during his stay if he could tell Michael what had happened during the procedure while the family surrounded him for support. The doctor agreed.

As soon as Michael came to his room he called me immediately on my cell phone. He wanted to know where I was and please come back to the room to see him. I figured he would be able to tell I had been crying and he would know something was wrong. I walked to his room trying to gain my composure. He immediately asked me, "Well, how did it go?" I told him we are waiting for the doctor to tell us. He should be here any minute. Then one by one the kids start coming into the room. They all gave him hugs and kisses and told him they loved him. He looked at me irritated that they were there because he told me on the way to the hospital the night before that he didn't want anyone to know he was there and he didn't want any company. It didn't take but a few seconds after they were hugging and kissing him for him to forget about that all together. In the end he was really happy they had come to see him.

Then, almost on cue in the room walks the doctor. Michael said ``so what's the verdict doc?'' The doctor started to describe to him you have a tumor in your esophagus that appears to be cancer. The biopsy will determine that for sure. The results will take some time to get back. We do have another test or two we can take but we couldn't do those until Monday. If you would like to stay in the hospital over the weekend we could perform those as well. As the kids and I waited for his reaction, and as I held him on one side, our son on the other and the rest of the family in front of him for support he calmly asked the doctor "Well can you have someone come get this IV out of my arm so I can go home?" The doctor said yes and left the room. Michael immediately turned to me and said,

"This must be why the kids are here, huh?" I said yes it is. He told us all very strongly, don't worry about it, people beat cancer every day. This was not the reaction I thought he'd have but it immediately made me feel better and the kids as well. We knew he's always been a fighter, and to all of us he's always been bigger than life, so although we didn't know what the future held we felt better knowing he had a positive attitude and would fight through it.

As soon as they took out the IV we left the hospital and went home. Michael was still kind of out of it and went to sleep because the anesthetic had really taken a toll on him. I went about researching esophagus cancer, treatments, life expectancy, and anything associated with it. I began a journey of learning everything I could about what we were facing and trying to construct the best way forward given the facts and the tools available. I also began researching insurance, cancer centers and what insurance they accept and so on. Our daughter, Christie, spent many hours researching, calling different cancer centers asking questions for me. She would come to the house every day for weeks to just sit and listen to me talk about how I felt, listen to me cry, hear ideas I had about the research I had done and also decisions I had made about insurance. I know she was there because she loved us and supported us but I also think she was there to monitor how I was handling the situation and to see if I was keeping it together. I think my mother may have also called her to monitor if I was eating or not. Christie was probably reporting back to Eden and Larry and my mom. I say that because I know they love us and that is probably what I would have done if I had been in a similar situation.

This is the moment that I feel so very close to any and all cancer patients and their families when they are told this devastating news with no experience of information, facts or options about the cancer that the doctor just tells you matter of fact that you may have.

This is the most life changing moment in a cancer patient and their family's lives. It is a pivotal moment that I must absolutely make this point, DO NOT GIVE UP AT THIS POINT!!!!!!!!! DO NOT THINK IT IS THE END!!!!!!!!! DO NOT LISTEN TO THE DOCTOR IF HE IS NEGATIVE AND A DOOMSAYER!!!!!! EDUCATE YOURSELF!!!!!! MIRACLES DO HAPPEN!!!!! HANG IN THERE!

DO RESEARCH! Get more than one and maybe more than two opinions before you make up your mind on how you will proceed. Many people give up at this point. Some of these people will end their life because they think there is no hope. There is hope!!!! Please do yourself and your loved ones a favor and start your journey with research and multiple opinions from different experts in the field of your type of cancer.

My personal opinion is when you make your decision on who you will use to treat yourself or a loved one make sure it is someone you feel very comfortable with. This is the story of our journey through the process after we get the devastating news of "Cancer".

*Disclosure: I am not a doctor and I am not prescribing any medical advice to anyone. I am only interested in sharing with others our story, both my husbands' journey as a cancer patient, my journey as a caregiver for my husband dealing with cancer and our family and friends' journey who are all victims as well when someone they love or care about gets this devastating news.

Chapter Three

Several days before Michael went into the hospital we had signed up for a construction project in an out of town location about an hour drive from our house. This project wasn't in the prospecting field, it was a construction project. A previous customer had called out of the blue and had another project available if we would like to perform it. The project had come at a good time as we were between jobs and in need of income. It would require that Michael stay out of town and supervise the project until it was completed. After this devastating news we had to scramble about how to complete this project. We have been blessed with a wonderful family that I am thankful every day for. Our son-in-law stepped up to say he could do the job with Michael there to supervise. He knew Michael was weak and could not physically help but he told us that he could complete the project with a few contractors that he could hire in the city we were working in. Our son also volunteered to help with part of the job that Michael would generally do which required heavy equipment work.

Day by day Michael continued to get weaker and thinner especially because his esophagus was becoming more blocked as time went by. In the meantime, I have been researching different options that people use to help them with cancer. There are many on the internet that sell different pills, and so on that promise to cure cancer. I wanted to tread very carefully. It was important to save my husband's life. Making a wrong decision meant losing him. That was not an option for me. That put more pressure on me but also made me more determined than ever to come up with a plan to beat this thing. I spent weeks, with very little sleep researching options, looking at what possibilities we could use until we talked to the doctor on March 20, 2014. That was the day when we would officially get the results from the doctor of the biopsy. I had called numerous times, multiple doctors and locations trying to get the results over the phone but they refused to give them to me. We would have to wait to see the doctor personally for the results. Waiting for the results of something like this is rough. We had to just keep busy working so the waiting didn't drive us crazy. Working on kicking this cancer's butt was priority number one!

During my research I had been impressed with multiple reports about baking soda. The reason this caught my attention is three fold. 1) There was one guy who had received a similar devastating report from his doctor telling him go home and take care of your arrangements. He explained how he started a baking soda protocol and after 12 days of taking the protocol the doctor told him at a scheduled checkup the cancer was gone. 2) A doctor in Europe named Dr. Simoncini had injected his patients with baking soda into their veins and he had very positive results. 3) Finally, and this one did the most to influence me or make an impression on me about baking soda. A doctor in the 1800's knew 5 sisters. All but 1 of them had died because of breast cancer. The doctor asked the remaining sister what she did differently compared to her sisters. She told him that she loved to eat baking soda and black strap molasses. Her sisters just would not eat it. The doctor found this curious and started using this approach over the years on approximately 200 of his patients that were diagnosed with cancer. A large percentage survived for multiple years and about half of his patients went into remission.

I had decided that this protocol was worth taking and it was economical. I went to the health food store and purchased Bob Mills' purified baking soda and black strap molasses. I must tell you that black strap molasses is not tasty. It has a nasty taste in my opinion and my husband's but when you are fighting for your life you don't care.

Our son was also doing research and had contacted his natural health doctor again and scheduled Michael an appointment with her. We decided to see what options she offered. We were on a mission to educate ourselves and determine the best way forward. She told us that he needed to take Aloe, Lugol's Iodine and to also continue taking Samento. There were other items she prescribed that we did purchase but honestly we did not use them.

I sat down with Michael and told him what information I had personally found on baking soda and black strap molasses and I believed we should give it a try and keep using the Samento and the Lugol's Iodine. Michael agreed. I had learned that cancer loves sugar and an individual's PH is important in the ability of cancer to survive and grow. A PH of 7.0-7.25 is a good range. 7.5 Cancer goes dormant. 8.0 Cancer dies. The way to check your PH is by getting PH strips that measure your PH either by urine or saliva. We always just checked the Ph of his urine. I ordered PH strips directly off of Amazon.com and they were less than ten dollars.

After researching the main survivors of cancer of all types, I found they have multiple things in common. The first thing in common was keeping on a high PH or alkaline diet generally consisting of a lot of green vegetables, and other items that keep the PH high. There is a chart online that shows the food that raises PH and the foods that lower it. Michael was unable to eat vegetables and was almost on a liquid diet. We could have juiced the veggies but he refused to drink anything juiced. So that limited our options to raise his PH. The second thing in common was their positive attitude, and determination to beat the cancer. If you believe that you are beat and the cancer is going to win then you and your body will just give up in my opinion. The statistics show that it's true. Your mind is a powerful weapon. Use it wisely.

News flash! Baking soda raises PH. So this was our option. So I created a protocol that we would use. A cancer patient will normally have a lower PH. Now just because you have a lower PH doesn't mean you have cancer it just means that the environment in your body is such for cancer to grow. Everyone is different so we had to find what worked for Michael. One guy on the internet stated how often and how much he used. If we would have followed his protocol it might have killed Michael. This was not the goal. We did not want to raise his PH over 8.5, this can cause other problems. We did have one episode where we raised his PH over 8.5 and we lowered it immediately with apple juice. Sugar lowers PH remember? Yes it does! That is good to know if your PH gets too high and you need to lower it. I can't stress it enough to try to never go over 8.5 PH. This protocol is actually a Trojan horse. The black strap molasses absorbs the baking soda and when you drink it the cancer absorbs the black strap because Cancer loves sugar. Then the baking soda is absorbed also which works it's magic in killing the cancer.

The other good side effect of the baking soda protocol is it did stimulate his appetite. Although he was basically on a liquid diet, for example soups, ensure, and cream of wheat, it was helpful that the baking soda would stimulate him to want to eat. This was important because Michael was 6'6" and used to weigh 275 pounds. He now weighed 185 pounds. His weight just kept going the opposite direction we wanted it to go.

Now within a few days of leaving the hospital, and after I had done the research and concluded to begin the black strap protocol with Samento and Lugol's Iodine, Michael went to Grand Lake in Grove, Oklahoma. Michael was needed to supervise the project that we had signed up before his hospital visit. Our son-in-law went with him for support and also to drive him because of how many pain medications he was on. Our son-in-law was also there to help supervise the crew, and to drive Michael over to the job if it was essential that Michael be there to solve a problem or answer a question that our son-in-law couldn't answer. I had also asked him to please monitor Michael and keep me posted on his condition, help Michael with his medicine or any other help he may need. He agreed and I felt better knowing that a member of the family would be close to help him if he needed help. I was a phone call away and could be there quickly if needed. When they arrived at Grand Lake they rented a little motel room that had a dock on the lake. Our grandsons also went up to stay with them on and off. Our grandsons loved to fish but they were also concerned for their grandpa, "Tapa" as they call him. When they were there they would keep Michaels' mind stimulated by talking about all kinds of things, fishing, prospecting, bigfoot and on and on. The boys gave him lots of love and they would help him with his medicines, black strap protocol, and preparation of his food. They helped him so much he gave them both nicknames. Daryn was called "Doc" because he would really stay focused on when and what kind of medicine he needed per my instructions. Bryson was called "Bruiser" because he was larger, stout, and Michael would say you will be my bodyguard. The boys took their jobs seriously. They also loved him very, very much. They would motivate him to walk out with them to the dock and go fishing, something that they all three would enjoy.

Every member of our family was rallying around him to help him beat this monster. He had started adding the black strap (what we eventually would always call it) for two days before he went to Grand Lake along with the Samento, and Lugol's Iodine. As he spoke to me on the phone on the fourth day he didn't seem himself. He described noises coming out of his esophagus and he was feeling rough and not quite right. He stayed in bed and really didn't make any sense. I called my son-in-law immediately to monitor him and keep me posted on his condition. I called my daughters and began to cry. I had been researching noises coming out of your esophagus and the results weren't good. I thought he was having the death rattle and he was going to die. Immediately my daughters drove to my house and picked me up and we drove to Grand Lake to see him. I was surprised when we got there. He seemed a lot better, stronger and he was even hungry. All of us got in the car and went to eat at a local café. We were excited to see him try to eat something more solid. Amazingly he did. Although this visit in the beginning seemed pretty scary it ended on such a positive note and with all of us feeling much better than earlier in the day. Michael enjoyed driving us to see him but insisted we go home, as he would always tell us all is well, I'm fine.

My daughters and I drove back to see him multiple days so we could monitor his progress, mood and just give him lots of hugs and kisses so he knew we all loved and supported him. These were fun trips and we enjoyed lots of laughs as he has always had such a fantastic sense of humor and on most of the days he was in rare form. His joking personality and positive attitude gave us all more strength to believe that all will be ok.

I still was curious what was really going on with noises coming out of his esophagus so back to the research I went. After researching other peoples' symptoms while taking baking soda I found that when you take baking soda and you keep your PH over 8.0, cancer will start to die. On the fourth day after keeping your PH at 8.0 the cancer collapses or implodes on itself. The research also stated to not keep your PH over 8.0 for more than 4 days. After 4 days we needed to keep it at 7.5. As cancer dies it releases carbon dioxide which is why they have the phrase, "How to kill cancer and not kill the patient." Fortunately Michaels' cancer was in his esophagus and when the cancer would die it would have an opening to release the carbon dioxide to leave his body safely. We believe that this is what was happening when he heard the noises coming from his esophagus. These noises would come out his esophagus throughout this process. I believed that this was a way to measure what was going on inside there.

During the time that Michael was working at Grand Lake I worked on insurance and our next steps concerning his treatment. The money we made on this project would help us with deductibles, co-pays, traveling expenses, and other unknown expenses during this period of time. We had lucked out that the government had extended the sign up time to acquire private pay insurance when you have pre existing conditions in 2014 to April. I decided since we knew that cancer is a costly disease we needed the best insurance we could get with the smallest deductible and out of pocket limits I could find. I had spoken to multiple cancer centers who told me they did not accept Obama Care but would accept private pay insurance. I decided to purchase a plan with Blue Cross Blue Shield of Oklahoma that was a Gold plan and would cost approximately $1,563 per month. We could not really afford this plan but we also could not afford to not have it. I purchased it in the middle of March 2014 and coverage would begin April 1, 2014. This plan had a $750 deductible, 20% co-pay, and $12 co-pay for prescriptions but most of all it had a maximum out of pocket limit of $ 2,500 and then the insurance company would pay all covered expenses at 100%. This is why I picked this plan. I knew that other than the monthly insurance payment which would be extremely hard to make, our medical expenses would cost us around $ 3,250 out of pocket ($750 deductible plus $ 2,500 in co-pays) and then the insurance would pay the rest at 100%.

Suddenly I get a call from Michael telling me he had a strange thing happen to him at a café during lunch with our son-in-law. He said an older woman came in with her daughter and although there were multiple people dining in the café the lady came directly over to Michael to tell him something that made the hair stand up on his neck, causing him to get emotional but in the end it really boosted his spirit and confidence. The woman bent down, looked him directly in his face, put her hand on his shoulder and told him that she was a nun and had been a nun for over 50 years and was retired. As her tone of voice changed as though a message was being delivered she said "there has been an intervention on your behalf and you need to hang on, you will make it through this health issue and your business will be very successful." Then her voice changed to her normal voice and she explained that her and her daughter love living in that little town. Michael was speechless, trying to hold back tears, he thanked her and she proceeded to go sit with her daughter and eat her lunch. Michael was blown away. He had just asked God to give him a sign that all would be oh right and then this lady comes in! Michael called me to tell me what happened and he told me when we went to see that doctor on March 20, 2014, he believed there would be no cancer and all would be ok. I believed he was right and we both got excited but agreed that he should continue on the black strap. He told me there is no way she could have known that I was sick, or what I was battling. This was the sign from "God" that he had asked for and received! He absolutely believed that. Our son-in-law witnessed it as well and also didn't know what to say. He just verified it happened and that he thought it was extremely odd.

On March 19, 2014, I drove up to Grand Lake to pick Michael up so we could go the next day to the appointment to see the doctor who would give us the official results of the biopsy. On March 20, 2014, as we drove to the doctors' office we were very positive but cautiously nervous.

As we waited in the doctors' office suddenly the door opened and in walked the doctor who had ordered the endoscope. He immediately asked us as he walked in, "had we seen the results?" I immediately stated No! I was a little irritated that he would even ask that since I had been trying to get the results for weeks with no success. Michael and I were sitting side by side and holding hands. The doctor sat down and said the results show that you do have esophagus cancer. He then gave us a copy of the results. He walked over to feel Michael's lymph nodes in his neck. Michael said well this is no big deal what can we do? The doctor said well your lymph nodes are as big as golf balls so I believe that the cancer has gone to your brain. It was like the doctor was telling us just go pick out your flowers. Again, so matter of fact with no options of what to do next or hope that he could beat this. I sat there speechless. Michael immediately stood up, stuck his hand out to the doctor to shake and said "Doc, nothing personal but I think I'll get a second opinion." With that I stood up and we left. As we drove back to Grand Lake we discussed what we had heard. Michael told me, "Joyce, people beat cancer every day. This is the second death sentence I have received this month. Let's just keep going with the black strap. What really makes it bad is tomorrow is your birthday, not such a good birthday present, huh?" I agreed but I didn't care about my birthday all I cared about was saving his life. I told him I believed that we would beat this. We needed to find the right team and the best doctors and I told him I'll work on what will be our next step. I left him at Grand Lake and I went home to research for our next phase of this journey.

Chapter Four

The real important question at this stage was what doctor or center to choose for a second opinion. I called and checked stats on all the cancer centers and read feedback from cancer patients, blogs and so on. How different people tried different types of treatment and what kind of results they had received. I was also focusing on the survivors, what type of treatment had they received that had helped them beat the odds. Michael was too important to risk his life with just anyone. A wrong decision was deadly, that is how I felt and that is what drove my endless research. I knew that there was a cancer hospital that was rated the No. 1 cancer center in America. It was located in Houston, Texas and that wasn't close but I contacted them and sent all the necessary reports, hospital records and film, disks etc to them for their specialist to review to see if we should come down for a second opinion. They called me back and said they do want to see Michael and they want to perform several more tests to determine the staging of the esophagus cancer. They had received a piece of the biopsy from the Hospital in Tulsa and would be running their own tests to confirm what type of cancer cells the sample was. We scheduled an appointment for mid April and they told me the amount of money that I needed to bring with us, deductible, co-pays if any, drivers' license and insurance card. They told me there were hotels on their website to help with our stay.

I called our kids and parents to update them on our decision. Our daughter, Eden called me back to say her father-in-law travels for his business and had points stored up at the Hilton hotel. He would like to donate them to us to use during our stay in Houston. We were thrilled to hear that so he called and made reservations at the Hilton hotel in Houston. He had enough points that we could stay using his points and our stay would be free. This was a welcomed gift. Eden had also been traveling for her work and had saved miles on an airline she used frequently. She told us she had acquired enough for two airline tickets and she would be glad to give them to us. I told her maybe we should keep those for later but I appreciated the offer. I figured we would need a car when we were there so we would just drive. The tickets could come in handy if he needed surgery or a procedure and was too weak to drive then at that time we could fly.

We were again lucky the money we made on the Grand Lake job would be enough to pay for the deductibles, gas, food and other expenses. We also had to expect that we would have to meet the co-pays until we reached our out of pocket limit. We were going to be driving near where my parents lived and planned the trip to stop and spend the night with them making it an easier trip and getting the opportunity to spend some quality time with them. My parents told me that they wanted to give us $2,000 toward his medical expenses. Everything just seems to be now falling into place. I was really overwhelmed that everyone was rallying around us. Our oldest daughter, Christie, told us don't worry about the house or our pets that she would make sure everything was taken care of. We knew this was going to be rough but having the support of our family helped us reach down deep and get the necessary strength to walk through no matter what challenges lie ahead of us. The love I have for this man is what would continue to drive me to find what could be the best way to save his life.

On April 15, 2014 we began our trip to Houston, Texas. About half way we stopped to see my parents and had a wonderful visit with them. They took us fishing on a dock that my dad had helped build and it was peaceful, beautiful and a welcomed treat. Michael really enjoyed fishing with my mom and dad and they were so loving to us both throughout the entire visit. I knew they were concerned and they loved Michael. It broke their heart to see him as sick as he was. Mom prepared Michael some potato salad which is his favorite and she blended it real well so he could eat it. She packed the potato salad, blackberries with cool whip and juice in a little zipped bag with a frozen apparatus to keep it cool. She wanted him to try to keep his strength up and eat if at all possible. He thanked them for everything they had done, told them how much he enjoyed himself and told me how nice it was of both of them. After hugs and kisses we were off to our next destination, Houston, Texas.

When we arrived in Houston, we checked into our hotel and began our stay of four days that would hopefully be the beginning to help us win this battle. We were hoping that we would meet professionals in the cancer field that were positive and would provide the answers we needed to beat this cancer. We were nervous. We had never been through anything like this and hadn't really known anyone who had. This cancer center was more like its own city rather than a cancer center. They do help you understand how to get around and our schedule has already been set for our time there.

The first day we met with a highly regarded thoracic surgeon that would tell us that Michaels' options were limited. The doctor told him he was emaciated and would not be a candidate for surgery to remove his

Page **41** of **209**

esophagus which he proceeded to tell us would be the best chance to beat the cancer. He told us that there are other options, chemotherapy and radiation. But first we needed to undergo some tests to determine the answer to what stage of cancer Michael had. The doctor told us because of the type of cancer, and where the esophagus is located that proton therapy would be his best option for radiation therapy because it would target only the tumor and would spare his vital organs, heart, lungs, liver, pancreas, aorta, etc. As he explained the advantages to proton versus regular radiation therapy we were in agreement that proton was the best choice for Michael. Although it wasn't the most positive meeting it sure wasn't like the last two conversations with doctors on this journey.

We also met with a dietitian who told us that Michael really needed to have a feeding tube placed in his stomach and that was not a big deal at all. This was the first time that Michael had ever heard of this, I had read about it but I had not shared that part with him yet. He immediately started laughing and telling the nurse that is not going to happen to him at all. I tried to explain what I knew about it but he just said, you guys keep saying it is no big deal but it is. You are putting a hole in my belly and into my stomach. I am telling you it is a very big deal. Even though it's for me to eat this is a big deal. He just told us both that he would not be doing that at all. During the conversation with the dietitian I told her that we had been keeping Michael off of sugar and trying to keep his PH up. She told us sugar doesn't affect cancer one way or another. Neither does your PH level. She told us to have him eat as much sugar as he could. I didn't tell her but I absolutely disagreed with her. And there was plenty of data out there of thousands and thousands of cancer survivors who kept the PH high by diet or other ways. There were many different studies that show that sugar feeds cancer. I felt we better stay on the path we had decided before we talked to her and keep Michael's PH up and stay away from sugar or anything else that would lower his PH.

The next thing on our agenda was Michael needed to have a breathing test and get some lab work done. The following day a PET scan was scheduled to determine if he had active cancer cells and if so where they were in his body. The nurses were surprised that his vital signs were extremely good. His heart rate was of that of an athlete, 57. His oxygen level is 99%. One nurse told him that was really good and unusual for a cancer patient. Cancer hates oxygen too. We knew the black strap was what had increased the oxygen in his body and his PH.

We had decided we would not share the black strap protocol with anyone at this cancer center. The following day we went to have the PET scan test. Michael said this was quite a test. You lay on a table and a technician comes into the room with a protective suit on holding a silver encased can that contains the radioactive dye that they will insert into your vein. He asked them if you are in protective suits surely this isn't safe for me? They said everything was fine and that after the dye was placed in his vein he needed to lie still for a period of 30-45 minutes while the test was being conducted. The radioactive glucose or sugary dye will only adhere to cancer cells in the body which will give a picture of where the cancer is in his body. Isn't it interesting to find out if you have cancer they need to put radioactive (causes a glow to be picked up by the equipment), glucose or sugary dye (substance that cancer absorbs) so the test can identify the cancer cells. That just reinforces my opinion that cancer loves sugar. And we do not want to give cancer what it likes. After the test Michael was told to rest and walk as much as he can the next day. We went back to the hotel after the test and let him get some rest. The following day after that test we didn't have anything scheduled so we went to the Houston Zoo and walked around. We enjoyed just walking around looking at the animals, enjoying the sun and each other. The fourth and final day we had meetings with the chemotherapy doctor and the radiation doctor. The chemo doctor would give us the results from the PET scan.

On the way to this doctor visit Michael told me to prepare for the worst. I did not want to believe that at all. When the doctor came in we both sat together again, nervous as you can imagine. The doctor began well yes you do have esophagus cancer. You can definitely see the tumor like an egg sitting in the middle of your chest. I ask and is there any other cancer. He responded with "No!" I immediately said "This is great news!" Michael said, "Well yeah but I still have cancer in my esophagus." I explained to both the doctor and Michael that I understand that but compared to all the possibilities that could have happened, brain cancer, vital organ cancer etc. Local cancer of the esophagus was the best news unless he had been cancer free. Everyone agreed. The doctor said I want to show you this PET scan; this is something I don't see. As he pulled the scan up on the screen he showed us the picture of Michaels body at different angles but he wanted to focus on when he went down the esophagus and could see the cancer at close range he described that this type of aggressive cancer usually has tentacles that reach out like fingers that are reaching, spreading, and growing. Michaels' cancer did not have these tentacles. Michael and I looked at each other and knew it was the black strap that had stopped the cancer dead in its tracks from growing and spreading. Remember at 7.5 cancer is dormant. We left that appointment excited that we were making progress and there was hope. The next appointment was with a radiation doctor. This doctor proceeded to tell us that our insurance will not approve proton therapy and we should just do regular radiation therapy and although there will be damage to the lungs and heart that is no big deal. We absolutely did not agree with her at all. We left to go home after that meeting and were told they would be in touch with us for another test to determine where the cancer was in the esophagus and how deep it was in the esophagus wall.

This appointment would be set for the end of April. After that test they could finish what they call his staging of cancer. The next trip we called ahead and booked a hotel located within a block from the center. This doctor would perform an endoscopic ultrasound of his esophagus. After that test was complete the doctor came into the recovery room and gave us the results that the cancer had gone through the esophagus wall. He also thought that possibly one lymph node might be affected.

When you take all the tests that were taken together it appeared to me based on the staging chart that Michael was a stage 3. After all these tests the cancer center never gave us an actual staging number. I used the different test results to basically stage it myself. Michael spoke to employees at this cancer center for the next few months trying to appeal the proton therapy with the insurance company. We both were under the impression that the cancer center was working on the appeal on our behalf. So we waited for them to call us back.

Chapter Five

We had continued to keep Michael on the black strap with every several weeks we would step him up to 8.0 PH for several days then back to 7.5 PH. His weight continued to crash and although the dietician at the cancer center told him he needed a feeding tube and I would try to mention it, Michael was not perceptive to placing that in his body at all. He would say, "You guys act like putting a tube in your stomach is no big deal. I think it's a big deal!" Until he was comfortable with placing a feeding tube we just had to work with what our other options were. I would try to see what had lots of calories but that could be considered liquid or close to liquid. Finally at the end of May, Michael decided he may need a feeding tube. This was good news. I was hopeful he could regain his strength and hopefully some weight.

Our daughter, Eden called around that time to tell us she wanted to take us both to Florida on a family vacation. She had a conversation with our daughter Christie and our son Larry and they were all in agreement this would be a wonderful family vacation if Michael and I, our kids and grandkids could all be together at the beach. We decided that it sounded like a fantastic idea. After that the kids took care of the details, they rented a house on the beach, we used those two tickets that Eden told us about earlier to fly to Florida for free and Larry came by and gave me enough money to pay up what bills I had that were necessary to pay and some pocket money for souvenirs. We were disappointed that our oldest granddaughter Carlye was the only one unable to go. And she was disappointed as well. She had just started a new job and was unable to get time off so soon. Because she had to stay behind and work she told us she would check our house and take care of our pets. We did take our pet Chihuahua "GiGi" with us. We did not want to leave her alone. I got the appropriate papers from our vet and she flew with us in the cabin in her carrier under the seat in front of us so we could see her and she could see us.

This trip was important to do before Michael would get the feeding tube. After the tube was inserted Michael would not be able to get in the water. The trip was booked and scheduled for June. We would leave on a Sunday and came back to Tulsa on a Friday evening. Michael was reluctant to go on this trip, and may have even dreaded it but I insisted that we were going and he decided to just go along with the plan. The moment we reached the beach Michael turned to me, gave me an incredible hug and told me "Thank you so much for making me go on this trip, I love you." My daughter captured that embrace in a picture and you can see what being there meant to us both.

Everything about this trip was perfect. Each one of our three children went out of their way to make this the most relaxing memorable family vacation we have ever had. Even our grandchildren were accommodating, thoughtful and wanted to do anything they could to especially make their "Tapa" relaxed and happy. The house was right on the beach. It was a big house and had a beautiful master bedroom downstairs with a fantastic bathroom with a sauna tub. We were told this is the room we would be staying in. That would be the beginning of this trip where our children treated us like royalty. I was extremely proud of the children we had raised, to be so thoughtful, considerate and to treat us with such respect. That's how they had been raised and it made my heart soar to witness it.

My son-in-laws would take turns making me margaritas constantly debating with each other about which one of them is really my favorite son-in-law. They both kept me laughing but also in margaritas. This was funny because I really didn't drink. Once in a great while but they were determined to keep me relaxed and having a good time. Their prescription, Margaritas!

Our daughters worked hard keeping up with all the kids, cooking fantastic meals from breakfast to dinner and made sure they had prepared what food if anything that Michael could eat. They constantly picked up after everyone, cleaning, doing laundry and driving us at times to and from airports and looking at the souvenir shops.

Our son spent most of his time working on attempting to catch the biggest fish he could so he could have his picture taken with Michael and the fish. He knew Michael loved to fish and to fish in the ocean, how fun was that. He made sure Michael had poles, bait you name it. He rented a boat and took all of the guys and the grandkids out to fish but they had no luck. He kept multiple rods out all the time to get this fish. Michael just enjoyed sitting on the beach with a rod, enjoying the beauty and the possibility of catching anything. Then all of a sudden Michael gets a bite and catches a catfish. No one could believe a catfish could live in salt water but he sure caught one. I got a great picture at sunset when it happened and Larry and Michael clapped each others' hands in a high five because of Michaels' catch. On the last day Larry did catch a smaller fish than he had hoped for but before he left to come back to Tulsa he had a picture taken of both of them with that fish. It was funny because it was small but it was still quite a memory.

This trip, having the family together (except Carlye), in a relaxed setting, with the beach a few steps away, a hammock to lay on, the sun beaming in the sky, watching our children and grandchildren having so much fun playing in the water, soaking up the sun, collecting sea shells, riding sea doos, finding starfish in the ocean, just every moment of this trip was truly priceless.

To top it off we were able to experience a rare opportunity when a sea turtle came up on the beach one night late and began to lay her eggs on the beach and cover them up and return to the ocean. This was an unbelievable lucky experience. The only reason we were able to know about it was happening was Larry had gone to the beach to check his poles. It was dark and we had been told that this was the sea turtles egg laying season. There were multiple nests throughout the beach that had been marked so no one would disturb them. As Larry walked out to the beach a couple that waited for a possible sighting of a sea turtle quietly told Larry watch out there is a sea turtle coming up to lay her eggs. Larry immediately came back and got all of us except Michael. Michel was too tired to go. The rest of us held each other's hands in a line as we quietly and cautiously walked to the beach and sat down near the sea turtle and let our eyes adjust to the darkness so we could see what was happening. We were all excited but didn't know really what to expect. All of sudden you see this sand being thrown in a circle violently around and around. The sea turtle had laid her eggs and was now covering them up. Wow what an experience to witness. Then she started back to the water. We got up and walked quietly in the same direction. When she almost got to the water we snapped a couple of pictures just to be able to see her well. It was dark and we did it quickly because we didn't want her upset or concerned for her eggs. She then went into the water and we went back to the house.

Michael and I both came back to Tulsa feeling wonderful about our vacation. We were both thankful we had the opportunity to spend time with our family like that and being able to relax a little bit was a welcomed event. Now we were ready for the next part of the journey.

Chapter Six

As soon as we got back home to Tulsa, Michael asked his pain doctor during an appointment to recommend a surgeon to place the feeding tube into his stomach. He referred us to a surgeon he knew and the surgery was scheduled in the middle of June, the week after we came home from the Florida trip. The surgeon we met scheduled Michael for the placement of the feeding tube the day after our office visit. The doctor could tell how extremely important it was to get him nourishment.

The day of surgery we prepared and arrived at the Hospital for Michael to undergo surgery for placement of his feeding tube. Because Michael had waited so long, and because his esophagus had become so blocked the surgeon could not go down his esophagus to place the tube, he would have to place it from the outside of Michael's stomach. This meant taking several cuts in his abdomen, one for the tube to blow up the area inside for the doctor to see and the other to place the feeding tube through to his stomach. This was scheduled to be an outpatient surgery but after the procedure was done the doctor decided Michael needed to stay in the hospital at least one day for recovery.

This surgery was rough on him especially because he was so weak. The hospital staff placed a cot for me by his bed and allowed me to continue to give him his regular pain medicine with nurse's supervision and with the doctor's approval. This was one stipulation I insisted on because I did want Michael to endure withdrawals or additional discomfort during his hospital stay. Michel was on an incredible amount of medicine and the typical pain medicine given in the hospital would not be sufficient. The doctor agreed so I was relieved Michael could remain comfortable.

I need to tell you that neither one of us was familiar with a feeding tube. We had asked many questions, we watched a YouTube video but it still does not prepare you with confidence that you know what you are doing.

A nurse was supposed to come to our house on Monday to show us how to use the tube, at least that was our understanding. The surgery was on Friday, Michael was discharged to come home on Saturday and we were anxious to get him going with his nutrition. We had to wait until Monday for the nurse before he could use the tube. And believe me Michael was very nervous about having this tube in his stomach.

We waited and waited until finally around 5 or 6 pm Monday evening and the nurse showed up at our house. She brought several items we needed with her and the formula for his nutrition had already been delivered earlier that day. The nurse gave us the syringe she brought, told us what to do and then she got up to leave. We told her wait, don't you need to show us how to do it, or watch us use the tube? She said no and just walked out to get in her car to leave. Michael and I just looked at each other in shock. Our grandson, Daryn "Doc" was there as well and could not believe it.

We all believed this was pretty important to not screw up. But with no real instruction that made you confident, we started to use the tube. I could not believe that a healthcare professional would think that telling someone how to use their feeding tube would be sufficient instead of showing or supervising someone while they use their feeding tube for the first time. I also thought there had to be certain things we should not do but we did not know what those were. Unbelievable as it was we didn't have a choice but to see if we could figure it out. I was mad about the way we were treated but I had to focus on Michael and figuring out how to feed him. The sensation was weird at first for Michael but he said it was good to feel full. He hadn't felt that way in a long time. That gave me hope we were making progress now. We all just grinned that he was now getting some nutrition.

The dietician that had placed the order for Michaels' food told us how many containers of the formula he needed to take in to be able to gain weight which was his ultimate goal. This would prove to be a constant battle for almost a year of on and off challenges with the tube and being able to feed him enough so he wouldn't lose any more weight.

Michael hadn't had the tube for more than a few weeks and all of sudden when we poured liquid into the tube the liquid leaked out around the tube on the skin on his stomach. We immediately called the surgeon's office that had placed the tube and the answering service told us to go to the hospital. We remembered the surgeon had also told us to go to the hospital if we had any problem so we loaded up and went to the emergency room. We expected to find professionals who could fix what was causing the leak. Michael was very nervous and anxious about this tube in this stomach falling out and having a hole there. After he was checked in at the front desk at the emergency room he was taken back to another smaller room to wait for the doctor. The nurse came in asking what are you here for, how long have you had the feeding tube, etc? When she found out that he had the feeding tube placed recently, less than 3 months, she just flipped out. She told us we can't help you with that. The doctor here will not even look at it. We asked her well where else do we go. Our doctor told us to come to the emergency room because time is of the essence so Michael doesn't require another surgery. She said sorry can't help you guys. Michael frustrated asked her "do I need to sign anything to get out of here" and she replied "no."

We went back to our car and on the way home in the middle of the night we called the doctors' office to explain what had just happened. The lady that answered told us she would have the nurse call us right away. We waited all night without a call. Are you kidding me! How scary is this! We had no idea where to turn if the emergency room couldn't help you. Who do you call? Where do you go? My god we thought this was an emergency.

All night we waited for the phone call that would never come. Michael was getting more anxious as time went by. What made it worse was he was unable to take his medicine or food because the tube was unable to be used. As soon as the doctor office opened the next morning Michael called and talked to the nurse. She explained to him that she had been on call and no one paged or called her at all. She told Michael please go back to the hospital and see the personnel at the interventional radiology department. Michael told her no I will not go back to that hospital and insisted that he wanted to see the doctor ASAP. She scheduled him for the next available afternoon appointment.

During the afternoon visit to the doctor who had originally placed the feeding tube, the doctor checked the tube and its placement and stated that the tube has definitely failed. He told us to go to the department in the hospital that the nurse had told us to go to and they would help us. He also told us time was of the essence so he wouldn't have to perform surgery and place a new tube in because the hole had closed up.

Michael began to share the horrific details of events from the night before. He described calling the doctor's office, following the instructions to go to the hospital, the refusal of the hospital to see him, the answering service telling him someone would call him back soon, and then the appointment to see him at this time. I told the doctor "I thought you told us it was extremely important that we get to the hospital in a hurry if we think the tube has failed?" He agreed that he had told us that and that time is critical if the tube fails so it can be corrected without surgery. He told us to go to the hospital and he would call down there and handle not just the instructions to correct Michael's tube failing but also what had occurred the night before.

We proceeded to the interventional radiology department and they had received instructions from the doctor and began to prep Michael for a tube replacement. After several hours of staying in the room waiting for the procedure Michael began to hurt because the pain medicine he took was wearing off. The hospital wouldn't give him any and wouldn't let me give him any either. Although Michael couldn't take most of his medicine in his tube we did have one pain medicine that he sprayed under his tongue. This had helped some but the hospital wouldn't let him have anything. We were again getting frustrated that he was waiting and now hurting and could not eat and we were again going backwards instead of forwards in his nourishment.

After a period of time, several hours, finally Michael was taken into an operating room to replace the tube using an x-ray machine and a wire to help place the new tube. It appears the technician would use the x-ray machine to see the wire as it is placed through the original hole and the existing feeding tube. Then the original tube is removed and a new feeding tube inserted and then the wire is removed, the balloon is then filled with fluid which helps keep the tube in place in his stomach. Before the procedure started and while Michael was getting prepped on the table,

Michaels doctor came down to check and see how he was doing. He was furious to find out the procedure had not been performed yet. Michael could overhear him shouting some very stern corrective words at the team that was supposed to have handled the tube replacement. In the end the tube was replaced with a new tube so we could go home. We were told the reason the tube failed they believed was the company that had manufactured the tube had a defective tube. There had been several other people who had the same type of tube come in that day with tube failures.

Tired but feeling glad the drama was over we went home preparing to use the new tube and continue to work towards getting Michael more nourishment. We were anxious to use it the first time but it worked just like it should with no problem so we were relieved.

It wasn't a week or so with the new tube that Michael began to have a cramping pain in his abdomen. He called his doctor and I called the interventional radiology department but they felt there should not be a problem. Michael was continuing to complain about the pain he was feeling. One evening he told me please take me to the emergency room because something is wrong. He had called his doctor and the doctor had suggested going to the one hospital that had refused Michael service because of his tube. Michael told the doctor he was going to go to another hospital. The doctor gave Michael his cell phone number and told him to have the attending physician call him and he told Michael about what tests he thought he should have and to have the doctor verify with him the results.

Michael did go to a different hospital, had a CAT scan of his abdomen and the doctor came in and told us that the tube is in the right place. They could not find out what was causing the pain so we left and went home.

Next day Michael was still experiencing stomach pain. He told me this is crazy. Let's go to another hospital so we did. At this time you could see his stomach suck in where the tube was placed and at the same time he would say it is really hurting. I would watch and it would suck more and more inside and then all of sudden it would pop out. While this would occur Michael was complaining oh my god here it goes again. When it popped he would say it really hurt. The attending doctor came in and we asked her to watch it happen. She called in a male nurse to watch as well. Neither one had ever seen anything like that happen. The doctor immediately scheduled Michael for a procedure in the radiology department so the x-ray technician could watch the results. He would inject dye into the tube and watch where it went in the stomach.

The male nurse came in and said the doctor was going to come in and say that the tube has been placed at the wrong location. We were relieved that maybe now they can stop the pain Michael is enduring. We expected the doctor to come in and tell us that the tube had been placed incorrectly and what they could do to correct it but that is not what happened. For whatever reason and we still do not understand why, the doctor came in and said, "Everything looks okay and you can go home." And within minutes we were discharged. Quicker than you could possibly even imagine we were discharged. We were shocked and disappointed. We had to go home again and more importantly Michael still had this phenomenon happening to him every few minutes. Where do you go if the medical experts don't understand what is happening to you?

Frustrated and getting madder by the minute he scheduled an appointment with the doctor who originally put the feeding tube in. During the appointment the doctor asked me to see what is going on. After he saw Michaels stomach sucking the tube in hard and then let go with a pop he was also puzzled. He said he had no idea why that was happening. He told us he would draw out of the tube some of the liquid in the balloon to see if that helped. He left the room to see other patients to let us wait and see if that helped. Of course it didn't change anything. The doctor came back in the room and decided okay let me put more water in maybe that will make the difference. He left the room and again no change. He came back into the room and said I have no idea why this is happening but I have other patients so I need to see them. Are you kidding me! Again, another dead end and no relief for Michael. He finally said if you want I can take you back to surgery and take that tube out and put in another tube like he had done in the beginning. Michael said you mean another surgery. Another two day event and two more days in the hospital and with little if any food, Michael refused to do that and we left more upset than ever. Not only did we not have any answers but the doctor seemed really not to care and was also confused why this was happening to Michael. It is scary when you can't find any doctor or hospital to explain why something painful is happening to you.

Eventually we decided we needed to see what makes it worse and what makes it better. So we began to watch after we put food in the tube how much it happened or when he was hungry how much it happened. It seemed to happen more when he was hungry almost as though his stomach was starting to cramp which would put pressure and pull on the balloon attached to the tube and when the cramping stopped it let go of the balloon which caused the pop. We started to immediately put food into the tube when it would start this movement. We learned that this would help give Michael relief. It was another lesson in this journey that we would learn with little help from the experts or so we thought they were experts. I do believe some of them were being educated at times right along with us.

Chapter Seven

Over the next several months we kept wondering what was going on with the cancer center in Houston and our insurance company in the effort to get the approval for the proton radiation therapy that Michael insisted he wanted. Every month or so some employee from the center would call and say how were we going to proceed and Michael would explain we thought you were working with our insurance company about covering the proton therapy. Eventually after several months someone called and told us if you want us to appeal to the insurance company you will need to come back to Houston, Texas to our facility and have another evaluation to submit the insurance company.

Here we go again. I thought you must be kidding me. All this time waiting for who we thought was working on our behalf to help Michael get the cancer care he needed and wanted. But in the end nothing was really being done or accomplished. We just couldn't understand how that could really happen.

Michael began to get worried telling me, "You know that I am afraid this is going to get the better of me if I don't get something done pretty quickly." He called and asked the cancer center again if the insurance company wouldn't okay it. What would be the cost of proton therapy if I paid it out of my pocket. You have to understand we couldn't pay for it out of our pocket. But if he could sell a claim or if we hit the lottery we could. The representative told him "$170,000." Wow, might as well be millions of dollars. We were unable to come up with that amount of money.

As Michael got more and more concerned I scrambled my brain trying to figure out what I could do. How I could help raise the funds. I had created a couple of funding sites that could help I thought but in the end they hadn't been too successful, they had helped but not what I had hoped for. So I was at a loss.

I felt heart broken. I was watching my best friend who would do anything for anyone in need, and now he needed something that I couldn't figure out how to give him. What other options do we have available? It was also again extremely important to not make a wrong decision, choose a wrong doctor, wrong hospital. I mean we had our fill with those decisions and this decision could mean the difference absolutely between life and death.

I changed my direction and looked at other proton radiation therapy centers that were available across the country. In Oklahoma City, Oklahoma there is a proton therapy center. I went online and sent a contact form to them and asked that they contact Michael to discuss possible treatment.

The next day one of the doctors called and spoke to Michael. Michael put the call on speaker phone so I could hear the conversation. The doctor told Michael since he had been diagnosed in March of 2014 and it was now October 2014 there was a one in a million chance that the cancer had not spread to the rest of his body. If this was the case they may not be able to help.

He told Michael that first thing he needs to do is schedule a new PET scan which can be completed in Tulsa for our convenience to see how the cancer has progressed. After that scan we can discuss the options available for treatment. He did not want us to get our hopes up because he had told us the odds were against us. We were devastated and scared about the odds although we were glad that he had called and he seemed to be knowledgeable and a nice doctor who would like to help if possible.

I immediately took the stance, no big deal. I knew this was right before the weekend and the PET scan was scheduled for next week so it would be a long worrisome one but I decided we would continue on with our black strap, baking soda protocol and believe GOD had Michael in the palm of his hand and everything would be okay.

The next week we went for the new PET scan. I knew Michael was nervous. He would try to comfort me and prepare me for the worse. I, on the other hand, was trying to keep him positive and keep believing we would get good results. These tests are ones that no one looks forward to. Not just because they will give the facts one way or another that can be scary but also the test itself is dreadful. Michael dreaded another IV the most. But like the warrior he is he took the test and then we went home to wait for the results.

I played the outcome over in my mind a thousand times. Always trying to remain positive even if I drifted negative I would try to stay positive. As in the past we thought the results would take days but the next day the doctor calls with the results. We didn't know it at the time but later found out when the results came in to the doctor office the employees there were all shocked.

The nurse had called and left Michael a message to call that the results were in. I had left Michael to visit with one of his best friends he had known since the 1980's so they could watch some old movies or just reminisce over old times. I thought this would be fun for a change of pace. I also thought it would keep his mind off of the call to come. All of sudden Michael heard his voice mail message alert him so he called back to find out what the message was.

As Michael called to see what had happened, you could have heard a pin drop. His friend said as Michael got the news there was a priceless look on his face, shock, unbelief, excitement, amazement, and feeling the blessing of God. Immediately the nurse told him "Michael, the cancer is only still in your esophagus. It has moved up some but not out or elsewhere in your body. We believe we can help you and we need to schedule you immediately so we can get your treatment started." Michael had also had this phone call on speaker phone as he had been getting hard of hearing and when both his friend and he heard the news; his friend just broke out in tears. It was an emotional and exciting moment. He immediately called me at work and I was frozen. I was in tears, happy, emotional, but just thankful that he was truly, absolutely "one in a million."

We were on cloud nine. We felt things were turning around. We knew we were blessed about the cancer still only in his esophagus but we felt this is probably how it was supposed to be all along. Had we gone anywhere else he would not have had the treatment he wanted or needed and more importantly he might have not been here alive at all. We also believed it was the blackstrap protocol that had kept the cancer at bay.

We scheduled the meeting to go down and see the proton doctor. We were also scheduled to see a chemotherapy doctor in the same building but with a different Health Care Center. We looked forward to meeting both of these doctors.

My parents called and said they would not miss this appointment. They wanted to be there to support us both during this visit. I thought wow my parents are in their 80's; they live over 100 miles away, I know they're active but what a trip for them to make for a doctor visit. They insisted on being there. We loved seeing them and were happy to spend what little time with them we had when they got there. As we all walked into the Proton center the women who work the front desk stood up immediately asking Michael's name, what doctor we were here to see and told us that they wanted him to be comfortable. They could tell he was weak so they helped him to a lazy boy recliner they had in their lobby and asked if they could bring him a warm blanket. He said, "oh my yes I would love a warm blanket." He was weak, thin and cold. You could just feel as we walked into this therapy center the air changed, it was an incredibly warm, friendly, loving place with people who loved working there and helping people deal with some of the most horrible and heart breaking illnesses.

One by one different people would come ask questions, have us fill out information but all the time allowing him to continue to sit in this comfortable chair covered in warm blankets. His comfort was paramount to their care. Watching how they cared for him with such care and love made me feel so grateful and hopeful that we are going to get through this. I knew we were in the right place and these were the right people to care for him.

Finally, it was our turn to meet the proton doctor. We were taken back to the exam room where they took Michael's vital signs, weight and so on. Next we met the proton doctor's nurse, an angel, who became an important person in this journey as well as she would coordinate anything the doctor or we would need. She spent time learning all the information that the doctor needed to know before he came in for the exam.

Eventually the proton doctor came in and we were so glad to meet him. He told us how unbelievable it was that the cancer had not spread. He gave Michael about a 40% chance to beat it which was more than anyone else had given us. I said 40%, no problem for a guy that is "one in a million." We were hopeful. He told us I will take you close to death and back, it will be rough but we will get through it. He explained the process of proton therapy to us and what to expect and how they would need us to come back down to perform a CAT scan with contrast dye so they could get the correct measurements they needed because they would have to build a mold specifically for his treatment. This process of making the mold would take about a week and then we could get our treatment schedule so we could begin treatment. The doctor also wanted us to know how important the chemotherapy doctor would be to this team. He stressed it would take them both and both therapies together if we wanted to beat this. Either one by itself would not work based on history and statistics. We understood and agreed. We had faith in this doctor.

I was still anxious about how we could afford it. I ask them what about our insurance. We have great insurance but what if they refuse to pay for proton therapy? They told us directly and with compassion, "Do not worry about that. We have a great team that does nothing but fight with insurance companies. You both need to focus on Michael's treatment." Unbelievable! Immediately we had a huge weight lift off our shoulder. We could tell this was a GOD deal. We were meant to be right here right now.

This whole process with the proton nurse and doctor had taken several hours and my parents were still waiting in the lobby. They had been chatting with several patients, read articles and letters from previous patients and were confident in the place we had picked. We told them what the doctor had told us in our meeting and we hugged each other just thankful that we had received such great news especially that Michael could begin treatment in the very near future.

Mom and Dad went on home since they had quite a drive and Michael and I went on to his next appointment in the same building to meet the chemotherapy doctor. This doctor we would find out was a great doctor as well. He was straight to the point, cautious and concerned about what was the best way to proceed and he took all the factors together such as the type of cancer to be treated, and Michael's state of health. This doctor would not steer you wrong and give you confidence you were in good hands. During the examination of Michael and his feeding tube, Michael told him he really did not want a port in his heart. The doctor immediately told him "oh we don't need to do that you have great veins." We were both shocked, again this was something Michael did not want and he was fearful of and came to find out he did not need. The chemo doctor began to tell us, there are several studies, trials and even historical numbers that show where strong chemo has been given to esophagus cancer patients but it hasn't improved the results any more than the patients that have received less strong chemotherapy. He told us what type of chemotherapy he felt would work best for Michael. He said he knew Michael was weak and the goal was to kill the cancer and not Michael. We appreciated that he was taking Michael's condition and well being at the forefront of his decisions. He also wanted us to know that throughout the process Michael's blood would be drawn and he would be monitored to make sure he could continue the treatment. He would coordinate with the proton therapy doctor for the best results. We felt extremely confident that we had found the perfect team that would proceed with Michael's best interest in mind. It was comforting to both of us to feel we had finally found a team of doctors who were concerned about his health, and that made us believe they were going to do everything they could do help him beat this cancer.

We drove home on cloud nine. We called all our children, friends and family and told them of the news, the treatment plan and how excited we were. Everyone had shared the disappointments, worry and wondering if things would ever get better and finally everyone could feel things changing wonderfully for the better. At least we had received some good news for a change and most importantly we had a great team and a treatment plan that would start in the near future.

Chapter Eight

We had only a few days until we returned for the CAT scan for the staff at the Proton center to take the necessary projections for the mold to be made for Michael's proton therapy treatment. Within a day or so since our initial visit I got a call from a lady at Proton center who handled the insurance part of the business. I was under the impression that everything was set to go but she informed me that we needed to go over a few things first. One important thing I needed to know was that should the insurance company deny paying for proton treatment after all their appeals we would be responsible for the difference of what the cost was and what the insurance paid. She wanted me to be aware of how much that cost would be. She wanted me to understand that they would proceed with treatment but would require Michael to sign a personal guarantee. This guarantee would be for the proton part of the radiation treatment. I was ready to agree to anything. Really how much do you think you would promise to pay to save your husbands' life or your own? She told me to wait until I find out how many protons will be used so I can give you the price. I ask her can you give me a ballpark?" She said I would hate to do that if I quote one price and it's wrong and let's say it's $250,000, I don't want you shocked. I need to get back to you with the correct cost. For a moment I thought oh no it seemed too good to be true. Now, we had a glitch in the plan. She said she'd call me back and I anxiously awaited her call.

Suddenly my cell phone rang and the caller id showed the Proton center so I knew it was the lady to tell me the dollar amount of the guarantee Michael needed to sign. I held my breath and she told me

$27,000. She continued, so much down and the difference will be split in 24 monthly payments. I was so relieved that it wasn't $250,000 or $170,000 or anything crazy like that. This was a lot of money but I felt we could live with this. No matter what we had to do we could find a way to get this done. I knew God would provide a way. And should she win the appeal with our insurance company any monies we had paid would be reimbursed back to us. She made an appointment for us to see her on the same day when we were scheduled for Michaels CAT scan. At that time Michael could sign the documents or guarantee, give her the down payment and then we will be set to start treatment. Hallelujah!!! Next step I had to focus on was getting the down payment together. We had multiple family members and a couple great friends that donated to the cause knowing how very important it was, life saving, life changing, and because this was more reasonable than what we had been quoted before. With Michael unable to work our financial options were limited. So unfortunately we had to rely a lot on our friends and family.

Everyone came through for us and with the down payment in our hand and excited to move forward we drove to Oklahoma City to get the CAT scan so they could make the mold. After that CAT scan was completed and the documents signed we only had to wait about a week for the mold to be made and the treatment would be scheduled to start.

The chemotherapy doctor had scheduled 5 chemotherapy treatments that would be performed once a week for 5 weeks. Before each treatment Michael would be required to get the lab done to see how his numbers were holding up and after lab he would see the chemo doctor for his physical check up and to discuss any questions or concerns he was having. He also referred us to a dietician that would monitor Michaels' nutrition.

The proton doctor scheduled 33 proton radiation therapy sessions that would be scheduled every day, 5 days a week, Monday through Friday, until they were completed unless weather did not permit. Once a week generally the same day as chemotherapy as well as proton therapy Michael would be scheduled to see both the proton and chemotherapy doctors for a checkup. Those would be long days which generally started at 4 am and ended near 6-7 pm before we would get home.

We also scheduled an appointment with his new dietician and this one we really liked. She immediately ordered a feeding pump machine to help with Michaels' tube feeding and we waited anxiously for it to be delivered. She had contacted the company that provided the formula that Michael needed and she ordered feeding pump bags, formula, 60mm tubes and gauze and patches that covered his tube. We also ordered a backpack to place the feeding machine and a bag of formula in for traveling back and forth to Oklahoma City for treatment. This backpack made his feedings much easier.

When we were notified that the machine would be delivered we were under the impression that the person that delivered it would know how to use it but that wasn't the case. The person who delivered it just gave us the pump and a set of instructions on how to use it. He apologized but said he had no idea what to do with it but he told us it comes with an instruction booklet. It took us a little while but we got the hang of it. We hooked it up on the stand that it came with and we sat it next to Michael on his side of the bed. There was a setting on the pump that would determine how fast the formula was pumped. We set it at 250. This meant it would take about 4 hours to empty a bag full with formula. A bag of formula would hold about 3 cartons of formula and water. If Michael needed 7 ½ cartons a day it would still mean over 9 hours of continuous feeding with the pump.

We thought this would work well during our drive to and from Oklahoma City. We could start the feeding pump while we were driving so Michael could get his nutrition. It meant more to prepare for the drive but it was convenient. All we had to do was just hook it up and let the pump do the rest.

Chapter Nine

The feeding pump was working well but Michael had begun experiencing panic attacks especially at night. We were so close to starting treatment but it appeared Michael was suffering a setback. He would panic, start walking around the room and then he would say let's go take a walk. He was panicked and felt getting out of the house would help. He wanted me to keep talking to him about anything to get his mind off of how he was feeling. This would happen over and over almost every day and night. Eventually when the walking didn't help with the attacks he would tell me to take him to the emergency room. Over a period of a several weeks or so before we started treatment we spent many days, almost every evening in the emergency room. They would check his vitals, listen to his heart and lungs, and he would complain he couldn't breathe. He was given breathing treatments and medicine to take for panic attacks. I think the worry had just taken a toll on him. I can only imagine the fear he never shared with me. I knew he was scared about the severity of his situation, his survivability rate, how he would endure the treatment he was close to starting and ever present was this incredibly hard to kill cancer in his chest that caused extreme unbelievable pain so he had plenty to worry about. Not to mention he was unable to work so he worried about that as well.

We both worked to get him through the attacks one day at a time. Then one night about 3 days before his treatment would begin out of the blue he got extremely sick to his stomach. He called for me to come into the bathroom and oh my god he was throwing up blood. Not just a little blood but a lot of blood. Because his esophagus was blocked and because we knew he was in trouble and unable to puke we opened his feeding tube and poured blood in a steady stream that would not end. I panicked running in place telling him this is not good. We have to go to the emergency room. My mind was racing, I need to get him to the emergency room, oh my god he's bleeding to death, and I better call an ambulance, oh god help. I told him shut the tube I knew he only had so much blood. I knew he was in trouble. He told me to get dressed and we will go to the hospital. He was calm how I will never know. I got dressed and helped him get ready to go and then helped him to the car. Every several minutes I would stop the car because he needed to get sick. On the drive to the emergency room every few miles he would say pull over and he would puke blood.

I had originally wanted to take him to one of the larger hospitals in Tulsa but I soon figured out we didn't have the time to get there. I drove to the first hospital I could get to. It was a small town hospital but it was closer than the rest and they had helped him multiple times with his panic attacks. We got in the emergency room and I told the lady at the desk he is losing blood and at the same time he went into the bathroom and puked up more blood. They took him back and got him a clear see through bag and all of a sudden like clockwork he got sick and puked up more blood. They were shocked; we were all shocked it was so much blood. It was then I realized that every time we stopped and every time he puked he lost that much blood. I thought he can't have much more of that in him. The doctor immediately got an IV started and gave him some medicine that helped the vomiting stop. I don't know if it caused the bleeding to stop but I think it did.

They checked the blood from the bag to identify where it was coming from and told us they were not set up for the kind of treatment he needed. This was a small town hospital so they told us he really needs to be transferred by ambulance to another larger hospital in downtown Tulsa for more intense treatment. Michael wanted me to drive him but understood this was for the best. I went to get my car and drove directly to the hospital just praying everything would be okay. I just could not believe we were just several days away from treatment and now this happened. I was wondering would this stop him from getting treatment. I was scared about what I had witnessed and was worried that this could take his life. I could not believe that we had been feeling that we were close to things finally turning around and now they looked bleak. I informed the family of what was going on and where we would be. They had received many calls throughout this journey when we had to go to the emergency room for various reasons but never because he was losing blood.

I finally got to the hospital the ambulance had taken him to. It took an hour or so for the hospital staff to locate him but when they did he had been admitted to a private room on one of the hospital floors. I expected him to be in the emergency room or prepped for surgery but that's not what happened. The nurses came in to get him set up with pain medicine and acid reducing medicine for his stomach which was given in an IV drip. Then a technician came in to get his labs drawn. She told us he must be having surgery in the morning because this one test they are requiring is for surgery or a blood transfusion. We just looked at each other at that news. I figured he might need blood because he had lost so very much.

In an hour or so the doctor on duty came in to talk to us. She wanted to know his history and she too thought there would be several tests taken probably in the morning depending on how his lab work came back. She told us that he would be given a floor doctor that would decide how to move forward in the morning. We could not sleep at all. We just kept talking over what had happened and how much blood he had lost. I knew he had to be scared, I knew I was scared. We had no choice but to wait until the early morning expecting that a new doctor would come in the room to see him, or we expected that any minute they would come get him for a test to be run, or a blood transfusion, or surgery or who knows. We waited and waited. Our daughters, Christie and Eden came to the hospital to check on us and decided to stay until the doctor came in. For hours we all four sat and waited and waited and waited. We kept asking the nurses where is the doctor? What is going on? And we kept waiting. Then in the late afternoon, the doctor walks in. We are expecting him to tell us what is going on but instead he walks in and asks us what do you want me to do? We all looked at each other and said well he has been kept here all night and day, the other emergency room acted as though he needed medical treatment, he's lost a tremendous amount of blood. Why was he bleeding and what's the plan? The doctor said well it's probably from the tumor or cancer in his esophagus. You haven't had any treatment so the tumor has probably affected a blood vessel in your esophagus. That's where the blood is probably coming from. You have lost a lot of blood but you are still a point or so from where we need to do a blood transfusion. All four of us ask questions like are you sure that there isn't a test to find why or where he's bleeding from like a CAT scan. The doctor just said no. He told us since his esophagus is essentially closed we can't go down his esophagus with a scope to see from the inside what is going on so there really isn't anything we can do.

We all wanted to say quite a few unpleasant words at this moment but I was just thankful our daughters were there to witness this or they wouldn't have believed me. Michael told me to go to the car and get out one of our syringes and bring it back to the room and we will use it to open his feeding tube and see if blood comes out. If blood doesn't come out we are going home. I went to get the syringe. Both he and I went into the bathroom to test his theory and no blood came out. We walked out of the bathroom and he told our daughters I am going home. I agreed. I couldn't believe after the scare we had the previous evening we could just go home. I also couldn't believe if this was the plan why we weren't told earlier in the day. Why did they wait until late afternoon. I guess what was actually going on was they were monitoring his blood to see if it dropped under a certain point which could take several hours to show up and if it fell under a certain number Michael would need a transfusion. It would have helped our nerves if they had just told us that in the beginning. None of us had eaten or hardly had anything to drink including Michael and we were all stressed, tired and worried sick. This was the hospital that had originally diagnosed his cancer. Remember the doctor who did the endoscope and how he treated me. We both agreed that we would never come back to this hospital. Michael told me even if I'm dying do not bring me here!

We asked the doctor to please tell the nurse to take the IV out that we are going home. We had treatment scheduled for a couple of days from now and really we didn't want anything to stand in the way of that. We had decided we were not going to bring this incident up to Michael's doctors in Oklahoma City because we didn't want anything to stop his treatment.

Finally we were on our way home from another emotional trip to the hospital with not much treatment or answers except from the initial small town hospital that had stopped the bleeding and had always been so good to help him through his panic attacks.

After we arrived home and we reflected on what had transpired the night before we decided we had a lot to be thankful for. Michael could have bled to death. That incident could have gone very bad. Although it was scary and it appeared life threatening somehow we were able to make it through it, stop the bleeding, and come home and be ready to start treatment in a couple of days. All we could do is just hug each other and thank God.

Chapter Ten

Now we have made it! This week cancer treatment starts. First day we travel to Oklahoma City for Michael to have a CAT scan for his proton team to make any final adjustments to his mold. They placed several pins under his skin to help line him up for proper positioning with the machine for his treatment that will begin the following day.

We were excited and prepared for what lay ahead. I knew that I was going to drive to and from Oklahoma City from Tulsa for at least 33 days most of them back to back. I also knew that Michael would have some rough days and I would need to monitor and encourage and support him going through this treatment. I had read many horror stories and his doctors had told us that it would be rough.

Finally the day we had been waiting for, the day is here to start treatment, both chemotherapy and proton therapy. We needed to be in Oklahoma City about 8:30 am. I needed to make sure we were loaded and on the road by 6:45 am. This meant I needed to be up by 4 am to get ready, get everything loaded, and get Michael up, ready and in the car.

Because he took his medicine every 4 hours and it was necessary to try to coordinate how to also schedule his feeding throughout the day with this treatment and the drive to and from, I would schedule to stop half way at a McDonalds to either give him medicine or food whichever was needed at that time. This would become a normal process during our trip. We almost looked forward to the stop. Sometimes we would even get out of the car to go to the restroom or we would get out at the picnic area just to stretch our legs. This broke the trip up for us a bit.

The first day during the drive I remarked, well this is day one and we are actually starting treatment. After today, we only have 32 protons and 4 chemotherapy treatments. This would become a daily count. Every day, only so many more, so many days or weeks down, or days to go depending where we were in the treatment cycle. This kept us thinking about what we were achieving instead of looking at the whole goal. If we would have kept focusing on how long it was going to take it would have overwhelmed us I believe. The way we attacked it, we kept focused on how lucky we were that he had started treatment, how many days we had achieved, what was coming next, and on and on.

Michaels' doctors were good at monitoring his health based on his vitals, weight and his blood work. Everyday that Michael was scheduled for chemotherapy he was also scheduled to get his blood work done. His chemo doctor would be able to check out how his body was responding. After his lab was taken we would be scheduled to see his doctor and he would physically check him and chat with him about any challenges he was having before we went to the Infusion center for his next session of chemotherapy. At times Michael appeared dehydrated so the doctor would add more fluids to his infusion session. These fluids to hydrate helped him feel better. I could see they made a real difference.

During Michael's first chemotherapy treatment we didn't know what to expect. The nurse that had been assigned to him for that day took him into an infusion room that had a comfortable reclining chair. The room also had a television on a movable apparatus that would allow him to see the screen in front of his chair. The nurse went and got him several heated blankets and several pillows to make him as comfortable as he could be. The nurse then explained to us how there would be several drugs that would be given before the 2 chemo drugs for pretreatment and these should help combat any reaction that Michael could have. These drugs were to be given over a period of time through an IV that would be placed in his arm every time he had chemotherapy. After the pretreatment drugs had been given, 2 nurses were required to be there when the chemo drugs were brought into the room. They would check that Michael was the right patient for these chemo drugs. I am sure this was critical to make sure a patient did not get the wrong chemo drugs. The chemo drugs were covered in a green bag which gave them an added touch of mystery.

During the first treatment, the pretreatment drugs were infused fine. One of the pretreatment drugs was Benadryl and would cause Michael to go to sleep. The nurse then told us the first chemo drug will be started slowly to make sure Michael didn't have any reaction but if he has a reaction it should be within the first several minutes of the infusion. The nurse began to start the first chemo drug and we waited hoping that he didn't have any reaction. Michael was in and out because of Benadryl. Luckily he went through the first 30 minutes with no reaction so the nurse increased the rate that the drug was infused. After that drug was complete the nurse started the second chemo drug at the highest infusion rate. She told us that he shouldn't have any reaction to this drug which he didn't. After the infusion was finished and the IV was removed which in total took about 3.5 hours we walked over next door to get his first proton treatment.

At the Proton center one of the technicians would come out to the waiting area and bring Michael back to a room where they had what is called the Gamma proton therapy machine. This machine is an unbelievable 2 story multimillion dollar proton machine which is very intimidating when you see it in person. The technicians that work this machine were very careful to help Michael through the process, helping him with his clothes he needed to remove and placing him in the mold that was specifically created for him. He would be placed in the exact spot that would line up with the pins under his skin. Then the machine would start up and lasers would circle the room and end up on the pins that were placed under his skin. The proton therapy wasn't supposed to hurt but

Michael did say he could feel something. What he felt we don't know. We assume it was the protons going in and out of his body. The proton therapy only took between 45 minutes to an hour.

We ended the first week with a great feeling of satisfaction. We knew now what to expect as far as the treatments were concerned. We had established a game to keep ourselves focused on one day at a time instead of the whole schedule so we didn't get overwhelmed or depressed. Our family and friends would call to check on the progress and to see how Michael was feeling physically, emotionally and mentally.

Second week started out good. My parents had driven up again for support and Michael told me why don't you guys go to lunch while I'm sitting here going through chemotherapy. I told him I will stay until they get you past your pretreatment medications and then we will go to lunch. Mom & Dad came into the infusion room and gave Michael hugs and kisses and words of encouragement. We visited with him for a while and then we left to go eat lunch. Before I left I made sure to ask the nurses to please watch him while I am gone in case he has any trouble. They told me if he was going to have a reaction to the chemo drugs it would have been on the first treatment so they thought he would be fine but they told me they would monitor him closely.

Mom, Dad and I had a nice visit. For whatever reason I just wanted something to eat that was quick, soup and salad I believe. We finished eating pretty quickly and went back to check on Michael. Mom and Dad were also worried about the toll this situation was taking on me. They were concerned about me taking care of myself and making sure I was eating and so on. They just felt a strong need to support us both because they loved us. This was extremely appreciated by us both.

It was a blessing that we went back early. I walked into Michael's room and he was white as a sheet with his eyes real wide. I looked at him and said what is going on! Nurses, doctors, and pharmacists were coming in and out quickly in an emergency type behavior. I ask him again what is happening. He told me thank god you weren't here a few minutes ago it would have scared you to death. My heart just stopped. What do you mean what in the world happened? He went on to tell me when they started the first chemo drug and he started to feel his chest crush and he began to get real hot and he immediately knew he was in real trouble. He hit his nurse button and when they came in they took one look at him and his face was real red they hit the alarm. All hell broke loose. The nurses immediately stopped his chemo and started giving him drugs to counteract the reaction he was having, doctors and pharmacists were called to monitor his condition to stabilize him. He told me you can't believe how fast they were moving, they knew exactly what to do to protect him. He was told that he could stop the chemo treatment because of the reaction he had if he would prefer. Michael knew the chemo was important and that without it they could not kill his cancer. He knew radiation by itself had a zero percentage rate of success. He told the nurses he would continue if they would slow the infusion rate down and give him more premedication. They called his chemo doctor to verify how he wanted to proceed and he agreed with Michael. Let's slow down the infusion rate and give him more pretreatment medications. They waited an hour or so to restart the chemo. Mom and Dad went home because they didn't think they could help and they really thought they were in the way. I just sat and stared at him as they restarted the chemo to make sure he didn't have any problems. I told him for now I wasn't going anywhere during these chemo treatments. Monitoring him was the top priority for me. I had asked the nurses, was there anything I need to worry about later when we leave to go home. They told us that he should be fine and that any reaction should be during treatment and not later on. The doctor made a note after this scare and ordered more pretreatment drugs prior to each treatment and the infusion rate to be lowered because it appeared to be what worked.

Finally he finished both the chemo drugs and we were ready to get his proton therapy treatment. Because of the reaction scare and the length of time slowing down the chemo infusion took we were running late to the proton therapy center. The infusion center kept in close contact with the proton center and they knew what was going on and about what would be our arrival time. When he had completed the proton therapy it was probably closer to 6 pm so this had been a long day. By the time we got home it would be closer to 8 pm.

As we drove home we reminisced about how the day had gone. How thankful we were that he had made it through all his treatments that day. Also that he lived through them. Although it had been rough he was pretty positive and looked way better than he had earlier which gave me confidence that he was going to be okay.

The rest of the second week went pretty much as we had figured it would. Since he had finished his 2nd chemo treatment the rest of the week was proton therapy treatments only. The actual treatment on proton therapy only would take less than an hour but the driving time back and forth made for about a 4 to 5 hour trip. As time went on each proton therapy treatment started to take more and more of a toll on Michael. The pain from the results of the treatment became apparent. The actual treatment didn't really cause the pain but it was the results. The proton lasers were targeting the cancer areas designated by the proton doctor and in turn the result was burning the lining of his esophagus and his stomach. At the end of the second week they wanted to perform a new CAT scan to see how the treatment was working. The doctor told us both that everything was looking great and that the tumor had shrunk in half. This was great news. It appeared we were on schedule and the treatment was also taking its toll on the tumor. The doctor then proceeded to tell us at this point that they will be coming down the proton machine and increase the strength of the radiation to really put it on the remaining tumor. This is the area where the tumor had started we guessed and it was supposed to be extremely hard to kill. We felt confidence in his doctors so we left thinking wow coming down and really strengthening the radiation. How is that going to affect him?   Michael was having tremendous pain in his stomach and esophagus area. Across his back in an area about the size of 8 inches wide and the total distance across his back was a burn that hurt him as well. He showed his back to his proton doctor and they gave him a gel that we put on him at night and the technician would put on after proton therapy. We were told not to put the gel on before treatment because it would cause problems with the success of the radiation treatment.

The first day of the treatment after it was coned down and increased a nurse had to help Michael out to our car which was parked out front of the proton center where I was waiting after his treatment. I could tell he was weak and barely making it to the car. I jumped out and opened the door and asked what happened and the nurse told me this one was rough on him. As I got back in the car he told me "oh my god I am in so much pain, please drive over there at the end of the parking lot and please give me some medicine." He was in incredible pain. We both were very worried that if the first treatment where they had increased the treatment caused him this much pain how he is going to be able to complete treatment. Michael even told me I don't know if I can do this. I told him it will be okay. I told him next time we will schedule his medicine to kick in before treatment and add a half or whole diazepam to help him to get through the treatment. The next day we tried out our theory timing the medicine to take effect before he went into the proton therapy. I held my breath while he was in there. At times we would bring our little baby girl Chihuahua "GiGi" with us so I would park right outside the door and stay in the car with her. She was very helpful with keeping him calm and me as well. Sometimes it would take a little longer for his treatment because they would put his gel on his back and as time went on and the weaker he became they asked him if they could help him get dressed. He would tell me he had to have some pride so no matter how long it took he would dress himself. He would let them put the gel on his back after treatment because he couldn't reach it. After this treatment Michael walked by himself to the car and when he got in the car he appeared in much better shape than the day before. We both agreed the medicine timing was helping make a difference. Thank God. That meant we had a chance to get through all of these treatments.

Michael was dealing with multiple challenges as time went on. One, his immunity was lowering because of the chemotherapy. This meant we needed to take great care to keep him away from anyone who could transfer a cold or sickness. This could create a back slide in his health and treatment. Two, the burn on his back kept getting worse day by day because of the proton therapy and that wasn't the only thing that was taking a toll. Third, the inside of his esophagus and upper part of his stomach which was being targeted by the proton therapy was being burnt as well as his back. This caused several other problems. He was unable to take on much formula because his painful stomach could not take it. We had to just work through it as best as we could and give him as much nutrition that he could take. As time went by and especially during the last week or so and several weeks to a month or so after treatment he could eat very little because of the pain in his stomach and esophagus. The doctor had told us it would take 3 months for the treatment areas to heal. This was a process we would have to endure and work through. We would see when he could eat more, feel better and have less pain as time went on. My biggest fear was that he was still losing weight. I just didn't think he could lose much more weight and with him unable to really take in much nutrition it was a worrisome time.

The five chemotherapy treatments, one a week for 5 weeks went like clockwork. The second one as we discussed was scary and the last one had a little scare to it as well. All of sudden Michael went white, started sweating and the nurse immediately stopped his treatment until she could check his vital signs, and take his blood to see if he was having a sugar attack. She started more pre-medications for the reaction he was having and after a period of time she started his infusion back up and he was able to complete it. Finally he finished his 5th and final chemo treatment. We looked at each other and were both excited. He was more excited than you can imagine because he hated getting stuck with needles, especially IV's.

As we started to walk out of the infusion treatment room the nurses all ran up and congratulated him. They gave him his very own cow bell with an inscription, a certificate of completion and then they asked him to come over to the bell on the wall and ring it to symbolize him graduating his chemotherapy treatments. He was thrilled. He loved the cow bell and thanked all the nurses for their excellent care that they had given him during his treatments. He had each of the nurses sign their name on his cow bell. As we began to leave he wanted them to know from his heart that each and every one of them is God's angels.

We had just a few proton therapy sessions left and he would graduate from that treatment as well. For the next week or so while we continued the last of the proton therapy Michael had begun to get weaker. His chemo doctor wanted to check his lab work to see how his body was reacting. We were told that he was dehydrated. The doctor ordered fluids to be infused every day until the end of his proton therapy treatment. Although he didn't like being stuck or IV's, infusing fluids didn't take as long as chemotherapy. Chemotherapy could take up to 5 hours and fluids only took about an hour and half. The fluids did make him feel better so they were really worth the effort. Michael could tell the difference so he was willing to endure it.

The last proton therapy session came and we were excited about it. His doctor told him how he wasn't sure at times if he'd make it but he was glad he toughed it out and finished it. Everyone was excited in the building. The proton therapy center had scheduled a luncheon for him with food and cake and a presentation of a really neat personalized coin that had his number and the Proton Therapy Center on it. It was very heavy and well made. He was also presented his graduation certificate. Michael went up to the podium in front of the crowd and made a speech to those in attendance. He told them how thankful he was for everyone who helped him from his doctors to the nurses. He told them that when you are given a death sentence and how devastating that is and then when you come here and are treated by such wonderful, warm, friendly, caring, positive professional people who treat you like royalty it helps you feel you can beat this monster. Everyone just clapped and cheered. Some people in attendance were in tears because his speech was heartfelt and if you had walked in his shoes or were a caregiver or had dealt with or treated someone that had received such news it emotionally affected you. It was a wonderful event except Michael couldn't eat which was hard for him but his doctor did have soup there especially for him. Michael tried to eat it but went to the bathroom to throw it up instead. After the lunch and presentation we went to the proton center for his final treatment. After that final treatment Michael was asked to ring the bell on the wall at the proton center to symbolize his completion of his proton therapy. We cracked jokes and laughed together as I stood next to him as he rang the bell with pride. We gave everybody hugs and told them how thankful we were for them and how much they mean to us and we would see them soon. He told them they were gifts from God, angels every one.

We left our final treatment reminiscing about how we felt when we started, the days that he didn't think he could make it, the scares, the pain, but in the end the success of completing it 100%. It seemed like a blur. I had driven almost 33 days Monday through Friday back and forth. Some would take 5 hours and others would take 14 hours. It just seemed like a dream, maybe a nightmare but we made it through. An important item we did figure out was using Benadryl with the other nausea medicines prescribed will help during chemotherapy when the other medicines don't help. Benadryl was very successful in helping stop the nausea.

Now we had to wait about a month to come back to see both doctors for a follow up while Michael began to heal from the treatment. We finished treatment on December 8, 2014 and needed to wait until January to see how successful it was. The next month was rough since his stomach was so sore and he was unable to eat much but we made it through to the one month mark.

During that visit another CAT scan was performed to see how the tumor had shrunk. The doctor told us that it had shrunk down to 25% of its original size and he believed it would continue to shrink. It did show that his esophagus had shrunk down as well. Michael told the doctor how he could hardly swallow water and the doctor was concerned that instead of waiting another 2 months to open his esophagus that he better schedule an appointment with a GI doctor to see if they could insert a stent in his esophagus. He sent the referral for us to a doctor he recommended.

Michael also expressed his problem with eating and the pain in his stomach so the doctor told him well lets cheat. We do have some tools to use if necessary. The doctor prescribed a pill called Mirinal that would help nausea, and increase his appetite. This drug is a derivative from marijuana but if it helps we were like who cares as long as it's legal. We got the prescription filled and went home. The next scheduled appointment to see the chemo and proton therapy doctors was at the PET scan around the 3 month mark after treatment. We were notified that the scan was scheduled for March 8, 2015.

Chapter Eleven

The proton therapy doctor had sent a referral to a GI doctor he recommended that worked in Tulsa. We had confidence in this doctors' recommendation so we looked forward to meeting this particular doctor. Michael also looked forward to getting his esophagus open. His greatest goal other than beating the cancer was being able to actually eat food again.

We anxiously waited for the appointment day to see the GI doctor. During the appointment we were told that first Michael would need to have another endoscope so the doctor could measure the size needed for the stent. Then the doctor would order the stent and should receive it in a couple of days and then reschedule another endoscope to place the stent at that time. We were disappointed that he couldn't get something done on the first endoscope so he could eat but we were willing to follow the doctors' instructions.

On the day of the endoscope, January 27, 2015, Michael was nervous that he would need to be knocked out for the procedure but he looked forward to getting closer to be able to eat. After prepping him for the procedure the nurse came to take him back and I went to the waiting room to wait as I had many times before.

I was nervous as can be. I just kept hoping for good news when the doctor performed the procedure. It didn't seem a very long period of time at all and I noticed that the GI doctor was motioning for me to come back to talk to him. I tried to remain positive but this appeared to be a conversation I would not like to hear.

The GI doctor proceeded to tell me that Michaels' esophagus was extremely raw and appeared burned probably from the proton radiation. He told me that until it was healed he would be unable to measure or place a stent in his esophagus. The best plan in his opinion was to give the esophagus another 8 weeks to heal and he would schedule the procedure again.

I knew Michael was going to be disappointed and told the doctor that but he reminded me that he did not want to do anything to harm him or perforate his esophagus. I agreed with him on that emphatically.

In a few minutes the nurse came to get me so I could go to the recovery area to see Michael. Michael was still out of it but was anxious for me to update him on what happened in the procedure. He was disappointed to find out that he would have to wait 8 more weeks to try again. I tried to keep him focused on the fact that this doctor had his best interest at heart. That he did not want to do anything that would harm him or perforate his esophagus that could create another crisis entirely. He agreed although disappointed and we waited until they discharged him and went on home.

Our goal now was to not focus on the 8 weeks but try to keep motivated so the time will fly by faster than slower.

We had another challenge that was starting to become more of a priority every day. Michael had been complaining about his left arm since about November 2014. The pain was getting more intense and he had a lump that kept growing bigger and bigger as time went on. His chemo doctor had the Hospital perform an ultrasound to make sure that he didn't have any blood clots and stated that it appeared Michaels' bicep has been torn. They had also tried an MRI but Michael was too sick for them to complete it successfully. The main reason he was claustrophobic and did not want to be placed in a closed MRI. The chemo doctor then sent an order to Tulsa to a place we were familiar with that we thought could perform an open MRI. Michael tried twice at this location to get the MRI but was unsuccessful both times. We just put that test off until he felt better and got healed from his cancer treatment. Since the first month or so during the cancer treatment Michael kept complaining to all his doctors and everyone who he talked to that his left arm was really hurting him. It appeared that it was getting worse as time went by. And his pain level was increasing to a point that his pain management doctor had told him we can't get rid of the pain only decrease it.

I told Michael let's focus on what is wrong with your arm. I made an appointment with a regular doctor that I go to in an effort to help him find out why he was having arm pain. I thought maybe he would be referred to an orthopedic doctor and maybe they could give him shots or something to help it feel better.

During this appointment the doctor told us "it is my professional opinion based on what you are telling me that you have bone cancer." He told us what we need to do is take some tests and one of them was an x-ray. I knew that Michaels chemo doctor had already scheduled that MRI that he had been unable to take so I stressed to Michael you are going to have to endure it. We need to find out what is going on in your arm. I called the place in Tulsa and they rescheduled the MRI with their head technician. They told me they had been thinking about how they could have performed the test since they saw him last. This experienced technician they believed would help Michael find a way to get through it. His challenge was they had originally wanted him to lie on his stomach but this was not possible since he had a feeding tube. At this time he was having another challenge because of his esophagus being so closed. He would need to get sick every 30 minutes to an hour as fluid would build up in his esophagus. This created an additional problem since he would need to be still for 45 minutes during an MRI. But we scheduled it and he finally made it through the test.

The results were sent to the regular doctor and to his chemo doctor. Our regular doctor called and said "It is bone cancer and its end game." Michael called me with again another death sentence. I said let's wait until we hear from the chemo doctor. The chemo doctor called and told us what the results said but he was like us and could not see how that could happen. We all knew that within a week or two there was a PET scan ordered that would tell us absolutely if and where he had cancer cells in his body. We agreed, let's wait for that test to decide what to do next. The chemo doctor did say he was going to refer him to a specialist for his arm, an orthopedic oncology surgeon. He would tell us more when we saw him at the PET scan.

Chapter Twelve

March 9, 2015 was the day of the PET scan. This scan would give us the definitive results if there were any cancer cells in Michaels' body. We were both a nervous wreck. My parents drove up to be with us again because this was a pivotal moment in our life.

We got up early that day because we needed to be in Oklahoma City at the Hospital by 8:30 am. We really had a hard time trying to sleep the night before. I kept playing over every possible scenario but I needed to keep telling myself and Michael that everything is going to be fine. We had immediately started Michael back on the blackstrap when we got the results from the MRI. We had been monitoring his ph throughout the cancer treatment and he stayed pretty steady at 7 or 7.5. All of sudden he crashed to a 6.0. This was when I knew we had to get back in the battle with our blackstrap. We had quit using the black strap during the chemotherapy and proton therapy treatments.

The time came and the nurse came and took Michael back for the PET scan. My parents and I sat in the waiting room for several hours talking and trying to keep our minds off of what the results could be. They could tell I was a nervous wreck and I could tell they were nervous as well.

After several hours I see Michael and he looks glad it's over but still weak. He came over to the waiting room and visited a few minutes with mom and dad. We then walked over in another part of the building because we had an appointment with the proton therapy doctor.

We left mom and dad in the waiting room and they settled in as they had in previous visits while we went back to see the doctor. The proton doctor walked into the room where we waited and took a look at Michael and said let me see this arm of yours. He was aware of the MRI results. After he looked at his arm Michael asked him "doc what do you think it is?" He responded "cancer". Michael said "why do you say that?" The doctor said "well, the PET scan shows its cancer." I think our hearts stopped, and I immediately asked, "What other cancer does the PET scan show?" I was scared to hear the answer but this is what we wanted to finally know. The doctor looked at me and almost shouted, "NONE." He told us no other cancer shows up, not even in your esophagus! He told us he wanted us to know he was dreading all day to look at this PET scan because he thought Michael would light up like a Christmas tree but this was unbelievable. It appears that the cancer is localized in your left arm which is rare and the chances of getting one but now two localized cancers are incredible rare. He couldn't explain why it happened but told us in the worst case you might lose your arm but not your life. That was a worse case. He was not an expert in that field and the doctor that we had been referred to was and he would make the call on that. He also told us that Michael would need radiation but that we could have that performed in Tulsa and use regular radiation instead of proton radiation because no vital organs would be affected. An important revelation was that he didn't believe we had any cancer cells left in his esophagus. That was fantastic news. He said it appears there is some residual radiation in his esophagus area and he told us he didn't feel that Michael's esophagus was totally healed. His expert opinion for the scheduled endoscope the following week was that we should reschedule for a few more weeks out. This was not something Michael wanted to hear but we were super happy about no other cancer except in his arm. We gave everyone there hugs and told them all thanks for everything they do and that they were all our angels. We also were thankful that Michaels' progress would continue to be monitored by both the proton therapy and chemotherapy doctors.

We went out to the waiting room where my parents were anxiously waiting. We took them to the side and told them what the results of the PET scan was and everything that we learned from our meeting with the doctor. We all just hugged and thanked God for this wonderful news. A huge weight had been lifted for sure. We gave my parents hugs and kisses and thanked them for coming and their support. They had quite a drive home so they were going to leave and we needed to go to Michael's next appointment with his chemo doctor.

The chemo doctor told us about the same thing the proton doctor had earlier. He agreed that it seemed weird about the 2nd local cancer and felt the doctor that he had referred us to would be able to deal with it. Both doctors really expressed how good this new doctor is. The chemo doctor was concerned that we had not heard from the orthopedic doctor yet so while we were in the exam room he placed a call to the orthopedic doctor on his cell phone. The orthopedic doctor apologized and told him that he would get us scheduled immediately so he could help Michael with his pain. The chemo doctor told him that he would make sure he received all Michaels' medical information and tests to help this new doctor with his treatment plan. We thanked this doctor as well and felt confident in our team of doctors that were in charge and would continue to monitor his treatment.

We drove home recalling the days' events and how lucky we were with the news. We thanked God that the cancer was localized but also that there were no other cancer especially in his esophagus or vital organs. We talked about how we were both pretty scared how the results could have come back and how unbelievable it was that we got "good news" considering all things combined. I just kept reminding Michael that God has him in the palm of his hand and he is that "one in a million."

We were now looking forward to the following week for the next endoscope with the GI doctor so hopefully the doctor can open Michaels' esophagus and measure him for the stent.

March 17, 2015 and this was the day Michael was really looking forward to. He just could not wait to get his esophagus open so he could taste and eat real food again. Or even drink something through his mouth. That is all he thought about. He knew if he could start eating that he would be able to get his strength back quicker. Since we had already been through this procedure about 8 weeks earlier we knew what to expect. We went to the hospital, checked in and Michael was taken back to get ready for the endoscope. I stayed with him until he was taken back for the scope. I went back to the waiting area and kept watching my watch hoping that it would take a while longer than last time. I figure if it took longer maybe the doctor was able to make some progress. But as with the last time it wasn't very long and the doctor motioned for me to come back and talk to him. Inside I just held my breath.

The GI doctor started to tell me that Michael still wasn't healed enough to open him up. He had a steroid ready to use and his smallest tool and he was unable to make any progress. He did not want to perforate his esophagus and neither did we. He told me if you want to find another doctor to try to open his esophagus up he would not have his feelings hurt because he just had not had a case like this. I ask him you mean you have never dealt with anyone with esophagus cancer. What he told me next was unbelievable. He told me that stents are put in patients that are terminal and they are temporary, they are not something that can be removed. Or he would not be able to remove one. He told me Michaels' case is unusual because his prognosis is good for the long term. He told me he did not want to put a stent in him for that exact reason and that he would rather take it slow and open his esophagus a little at a time. He said it was his opinion to wait another 8 weeks and he would try to open his esophagus with the steroid as much as he could. Then he believed we may have to keep this process up every 4 weeks until he has it opened all the way up or as far as he can. I thought this was an excellent idea and I was happy to hear that Michael had a good prognosis and I was thankful that he had not been able to place a stent. We wanted a permanent solution not a temporary one. We knew the stent had a lot of side effects so this was probably a blessing in disguise. I really could feel that God was keeping

Michael in the palm of his hand and protecting him throughout this whole process. I told the doctor that we did not want to change doctors. He had been highly recommended by the doctors' we trusted and since he was also concerned about Michaels' survivability and not making a mistake I told him that we both felt confident in his plan and his expertise. He thanked me for that and we agreed to schedule the next endoscope to try to open his esophagus 8 weeks from today.

When I went back to see Michael in recovery he was out of it but was curious how it went. Although I knew he wouldn't remember what I said I told him what the doctor and I had discussed. I knew he was disappointed but I really needed to get him to understand how great the news was although it was also bad. After he was released and we went home we went over the conversation with the doctor again. He then started to understand how wonderful the news was. He understood that him not getting a stent was a blessing and that if we followed the doctors' advice and moved slowly it was possible that he could have a long term solution that will benefit him much more and he could possibly eat more of the foods that he missed compared to the stent. We had other challenges to tackle so we changed our focus on those hoping this 8 week period would go by fast.

Chapter Thirteen

The next day we were scheduled to see the orthopedic oncology doctor, March 18, 2015. This doctor has an office in Oklahoma City and Tulsa so we were scheduled to see him in Tulsa. Michael's pain was getting out of control. His pain doctor had increased his meds as much as he could. The pain doctor had added a strong pain spray that is sprayed under the tongue. This spray is typically used on cancer patients and is extremely expensive. Thank God our insurance company paid for it or we could not have afforded it at all. The pain doctor went out of his way to make sure Michael was as comfortable as we could get him. Without him I don't know how Michael could have stood the pain. Even with the increase to the maximum dosage of his pain medicine the pain would not totally go away. Michael would just shut his eyes and rock back and forth trying to deal with the pain. It just broke my heart to see him in such pain but I was helpless to stop it.

I had become a distributor of essential oils. The funny thing is I had been taking a capsule that had frankincense in it and one day I looked in the mirror and noticed that this fatty tumor that I had on my eyebrow had seemed to shrink. I had been to several doctors and had an MRI and they told me I could have it removed but it was just a fatty tumor not cancerous. I hated how it looked and felt but I was shocked that it appeared to be shrinking. I looked up the ingredients in the capsule I was taking and I read about frankincense. It was thought it could help cancer but also inflammation. Believe me those who have dealt with cancer are willing to try anything. I showed Michael what was happening to my fatty tumor and I told Michael let's try it on your arm.

We had been trying heat or ice, this kind of wrap or that kind of wrap. We took off the wrap and I put a good amount of frankincense oil directly on the skin that covered the tumor. There was no confusion where it was because the tumor had grown to a point where it looked like a baseball inside his left arm. As soon as I put the frankincense on the skin and went and sat down, Michael told me he could feel it going through his skin into his arm. It felt good, he told me. After a day or so his tumor appeared to go down in size. It appeared to help the pain some but he was still in a great deal of pain. I kept putting the oil over his tumor. I had also emailed a couple of pictures of his arm to the orthopedic doctor hoping that they would get him in for an appointment as fast as possible. This became the best way to get information to or from the doctor by his head nurse.

The day came to see the orthopedic doctor. We were hoping that we could get Michael some immediate relief. The doctor came highly recommended but we were also very worried about what he might say. Michael's main concern was he might lose his arm. I had reminded him that if we were given the option of his arm or his life we were going to pick his life. There were other options for his arm, prosthesis etc. None of these he liked but he agreed that his life was more important.

The doctor after looking at the MRI and examining his arm told us that he felt that he could treat the cancer with radiation only. That within 2 days of radiation the pain would decrease significantly. He didn't believe Michael needed surgery or would lose his arm. This was all good news. We wanted to know how fast they could schedule the radiation. Pain relief was our first priority. The doctor told us "first we need to find out what cancer this is and where it came from." That meant we would need to drive to a hospital in Edmond Oklahoma and get a biopsy of his arm. The pathologists that worked with this doctor could determine the answers to those questions. Then within a couple of days of the results Michael could start radiation. This is not what we needed to hear. It would be days maybe a week or more before Michael could get any relief from the pain. With no other choice we went home disappointed but reminding ourselves we are closer and closer to getting it taken care of it. We also kept focused on the good news that he would not lose his arm.

We waited for another week until we could get the biopsy. The staff let me stay in the room while the biopsy was performed. The technician put a needle in his arm that had the ability to cut some tissue.

This was done after the area where the needle was going to be placed was deadened. While the technician was watching an x-ray machine showing where the needle was located in his arm he performed the biopsy. It was pretty interesting to watch. Another team of technicians were in the room to take the samples from the biopsy and look under the microscope to see if they were good samples. After they were confident that the samples from the biopsy were good then they told us that's all we need. This process didn't take long. We were told by the people in the room that the results would take 2-3 days or up to a week.

We went home and waited and waited. 3 days went by and then a week. I called and said this is ridiculous what is going on. The doctor's nurse called to tell me that the problem they were having was that the 5 pathologists that were determining what kind of cancer this was could not agree. They could not reach a mutual agreement and until they did we could not move forward. Several of them thought it was esophagus cancer and the others thought it was a new cancer. I understood why getting this correct was important but I also understood how much pain Michael was in.

We waited several more days and I was just done waiting. I emailed the nurse and told her, "This waiting is becoming torturous to Michael. We know its cancer and we know you are going to treat it with radiation. Why can't we go ahead and schedule the radiation so Michael can get some relief?" I told her other things which included I appreciated them wanting to proceed cautious and get this right but his pain was overwhelming. I sent this email around 10 pm at night. To my surprise before 11 pm I got a response from the nurse that she would forward my email to the doctor.

The next morning I was awakened by my cell phone ringing and it was the doctors' office. The nurse told me, Joyce, the doctor agrees with you and does not want to wait anymore. We want to schedule Michael for surgery next Tuesday to remove the tumor. She further told me we need to be in Oklahoma City to see them Monday before 11 am to get all the necessary paperwork and tests completed so the surgery could be done Tuesday. Michael overheard what we were saying and immediately said what and I gave him my phone and the nurse explained to him what the plan was. He was nervous about surgery but said ok we will be there. One more thing she told him, the last MRI you had done was not good quality. We need an updated one before Monday. She would schedule one at a hospital downtown for the next day, Good Friday. We agreed and he hung up the phone.

Michael was nervous, he was afraid; as he thought more about the surgery he couldn't help but worry he might possibly lose his arm. I felt the doctor would do everything possible to make sure that didn't happen but I also knew it had to weigh heavy on Michael's mind. The other challenge was the hospital we needed to go to was the same hospital that we had swore we would never go back to again. I just said we need to get this test done even though we are not happy about it. Michael agreed but remember he had many issues with MRI's and now his esophagus was even more closed and he had to throw up more often which will make this test even harder for him to endure. But he agreed that he would give it his best try.

The next day, Good Friday, the test had been scheduled at 7 pm that evening. We showed up as instructed and immediately were reminded as to why we did not like this hospital. The lady in the check in area came out and told us do you have his current lab work? I told her that no one told me to bring current lab work. She said, well if he doesn't have current lab work in the last 30 days we will have to put in an IV and get blood work or we won't be able to do this test. I told her we have to have this test. He has surgery next week and we have to give it to his doctor Monday morning. I told her where he had received his most recent lab work but of course it is late on a Friday night and they weren't open. She went to see if she could contact them but was unable. She then came back to tell us we will have to start an IV and do the blood work before the test. I told her to do what you have to do for this test to be done. She then proceeded to tell me your insurance isn't going to pay for this blood test probably and you will get the bill. I told her fine just do the test! It appeared she really wanted us to just go home and not do this test at all. Wow I didn't know how right I really was.

She took Michael back to a room to get ready for the test so he could change clothes. I went with him to help him change. He couldn't use his left arm at all so he really needed help with everything but especially changing clothes. After he was prepared we walked out and he laid down on the bed per her instructions. There was a guy there that Michael asked if they had a warm blanket because he was so cold. This man was very nice and went to retrieve a warm blanket to cover him with. Michael thanked him and apologized that these guys had to work on Good Friday. This guy left the area because his shift was over we assume. The lady who had been so rude continued to be very short with everything she said to us. Finally a nice little oriental lady came in to place the IV in Michaels arm. Now if he was going to have an MRI with contrast he needed an IV anyway. The rude lady asked the lab lady can you please draw his blood. The lab lady and the rude lady went back and forth for 5 minutes with this conversation. The lab lady said I do not have an order for that. The rude lady would say without the blood drawn I don't need the IV because I can't do this test. The lab lady said why don't you draw the blood. The rude lady, I don't do that.

Finally the lab lady tried to pull blood out of the IV with no success. Michael said please just draw the blood and he told her to use a certain type of needle. After minutes of the rude lady going on and on and this nice little lab lady could see I believed how rude she was so she reversed her decision probably against policy and finally she just drew the blood. I asked the rude lady so the doctor did not order the lab work. She just kind of shrugged her shoulders. That was it for me. I looked at her real direct and real stern and said, "Monday when we see the doctor I will make sure to tell him that he better make sure to order labs when he orders an MRI at this hospital so this doesn't happen again." The rude lady immediately checked her attitude and said oh no he sent the order. My thoughts were then why the hell are we having this kind of drama! It appeared through this whole process what she really wanted us to do was to get frustrated and mad and to just get up and say never mind and leave. When she walked off once out of ear shot I reminded Michael, "I know she is being as rude as she can and she really wants us to leave but we absolutely need to get this test done." He agreed and told me he would do his best.

When she came back she asked me to see where the area we are testing is located. Michael showed her the large lump in his arm. She wanted to move his arm and Michael told her I can't move my arm and it is extremely painful. She then rudely said "I don't know what kind of results we are going to get because if I can't get you in a certain position this test will not be able to get to that area. I looked at her trying to keep my composure just as I had asked Michael to do and I said "Look do the best you can the doctor is well aware of his limitation and he is aware he can't move his arm and he is the one who scheduled this test!"

The rude lady didn't respond and went about to process Michaels' blood through some machine in the room we were in to see if Michaels' levels were where they had to be so we could move forward with this test. She was clearly frustrated and was hoping that his levels were too low but they were fine and she would have to perform the test. You could tell this wasn't what she wanted. I just couldn't figure out why she had such a poor attitude and why she was trying to treat us so poorly. Was it because she had to work on Good Friday? Michael had even apologized to her for that. Was it a full moon? Was it she didn't want to be here? Michael didn't want to be here either but he didn't really have a choice. She could just quit and go home if she didn't like her job. Then I thought every time we come to this hospital they treat us horribly. Is there something written on his chart that makes them act that way. I didn't know. I just knew that I would share this experience with the doctor on Monday and let them know what terrible treatment we received. I knew once we got through this test we would never come back to this hospital, ever! I kept thinking I hope she never is frail and in need of others to treat her for any medical condition and if so I hope she doesn't get a person like her. There should be some standard of care for people with at least some level of respect. This lady was definitely lacking in all those areas.

She told me I could wait in the closet type room where Michael changed his clothes as she started rolling the bed Michael was laying on toward the room to perform the MRI, I could clearly see the room from where I stood. I went to the little room as she instructed me and I heard Michael ask her "could I please get another warm blanket if I'm cold?" She just scolded him and told him "No! I can't leave here." I thought wow what a terribly rude heartless woman. How she got or kept her job was beyond me. I felt so sorry for Michael. I could just feel his pain and fear with this woman being in charge of this test. This was just the beginning of this nightmare.

She rolled Michael into the room and tried to position him for the test. I heard Michael moan and tell her that he couldn't put his arm in certain ways. It hurt too much. All of a sudden she came to where I was sitting and asked me to come help her with him. I walked over to the room he was in and she instructed me I could come to the door but not past the door. The door was open so Michael could see me. He asked me to go get him one of his pain sprays and I quickly did just exactly as he asked. The lady pulled him out of the room to take his pain spray then rolled him back in. As I stood there giving Michael moral support to hang in there it appeared this also caused this rude lady to be nicer and less rough with him. He eventually was placed in the position she was happy with and he thought he could hold. When she said ok we are ready to proceed. He asked for a small towel to be placed over his face so he wouldn't see that he was in a tight space when she slid him into the MRI machine. She put the towel over his face and then she shut his door. Before she shut the door she told him she could hear him and that she would talk him through the test. I told him I am right here honey please just hang in there. I just hoped it gave him comfort knowing that I was right outside that door watching what was going on.

Outside the door was a panel that showed pictures of his arm area during the test. It was amazing to me that you could see the area the doctor wanted pictures of. I waited on the outside of the door sitting by her as she ran several minutes of different views of his arm in this test. She would tell him this one is so many minutes long etc. I just kept almost holding my breath knowing how hard it must be in there for him. Finally the test was over. I breathed a sigh of relief. And I know that Michael was clearly happy to have made it through it. The lady rolled him out of the room and left him in the middle of the walk way of the room to take his IV out. I walked over to him and she asked if he needed any help. I told her no I will help him get to the room and change. Thank you anyway. I grabbed Michael and helped him to the changing room and helped him get his clothes changed. He whispered to me, "Oh my god she was torturing me." I told him I know let's just get out of here. As soon as he was dressed we walked out the door and as far away from that lady as we could get. As horrible as she was I will say there was one employee there that checked us in, a very nice guy that told me if you really need a copy of the disc to take to your doctor for Monday I will come up here tomorrow even though it is my day off and I will make you a copy. I thanked him very much, gave him my cell phone number and told him please call me tomorrow when you have it ready and I will pick it up. I was pleased that he did exactly what he promised and I was able to get the MRI disc so we were able to take it to Michaels' doctor on Monday.

The rest of the weekend went reasonably quick. I was busy making sure I would pack everything we needed to get through the several days we would be in Oklahoma City. Other than the normal items that needed packing, I needed to make sure we had enough formula, water to mix with the formula and medicine and all of his medicines. Every day I mixed up 24 hours worth of medicines into water bottles. Since all of his medicine needed to be crushed each dose was placed into a small amount of water in a water bottle. This way the medicine would be good and dissolved to pass quickly and without clogging his feeding tube. I had to make sure to schedule all of these items. Monday morning when we left I needed to make sure I did not forget anything at all. I also mixed up several formula containers with water in water bottles. This was the best way to mix his nutrition to make it easier for us to give it to him during the next day. We had learned this trick during the cancer treatment trips to Oklahoma City.

Monday morning came and we were loaded up and ready to go. Both of us were more than ready for Michael to get some pain relief. We followed the instructions to the doctors' office in Oklahoma City and had a pretty good time. During the doctor visit he looked at the current MRI and told us it was much better quality than the first. He spent some time explaining what he hoped to achieve which was to remove the tumor mass in Michael's arm without disturbing the nerves, blood vessels, tendons and so on. He warned us that if he got into Michaels' arm and was unable to remove it at least he could get a piece of it for another biopsy. Then he would close his arm and we would have to wait 3 more weeks for the surgery to heal before Michael could start radiation. We told the doctor my god we hope that he could remove the tumor. For Michael to wait 3 more weeks for Michael to get any kind of relief from the pain was more than we could imagine. The doctor could tell the pain was taking an incredible toll on him. That is why he had decided to proceed with this surgery anyway. We told him we had tremendous confidence in his ability and then left to follow his instructions to go to the hospital where the procedure was going to be performed.

It was necessary for Michael to get some labs and an EKG done as a precaution before surgery. We also had to fill out the necessary paperwork for the hospital, insurance information, driver license, etc. We were then told to be back to the hospital by 5 am in the morning for surgery prep. Surgery is scheduled for 7 am in the morning.

We were tired. I hadn't slept the night before because I was too worried that I would over sleep and we would be late. After the drive, the appointments and the tests we were really tired. On top of that I had not been able to eat. I made sure Michael had his nutrition and I drank a coffee or two but I just didn't want to take any time to eat and I also hated eating in front of him unless I just had to. This gave me a headache and I was getting a little agitated. I just wanted to eat and go to sleep.

Next thing on our agenda was to find a hotel. The place that the doctor office recommended would not work because we were not fond of the location. We decided to get on the highway and go toward an area of the city we were familiar with. About 8 miles or so we saw a Best Western sign. That made our decision easy. We knew immediately this is where we were going to stay. I figured we probably would not be leaving once we got to our room so before we checked in and with Michaels insistence I went through a Starbucks to get a couple of grilled cheese sandwiches, a lemon pound cake and a drink. I knew I could put one sandwich in the refrigerator in our room and heat it up later if I got hungry.

We then checked in to our hotel. I unloaded the car so we could get comfortable. Michael went to get ice and a couple of diet cokes for the refrigerator for later if I needed them. After all that was completed and Michael took his medicine we laid down to take a well needed nap. It was late afternoon and we were tired. To be at the hospital by 5 am in the morning we would need to be up by 3 am. I knew that I would probably have to reload most of our belongings even though we had rented the room for 2 nights. I just couldn't leave his medicine and other items in the room. We took a nap but the pain Michael was in made it impossible for either one of us to sleep very long. Every 3 hours he would ask me when he could take his medicine. Sometimes he would ask every 2 hours. The pain was overwhelming. We knew we were hours away of what we hoped would be some pain relief for him. The one thing the doctor did tell us is that he planned to do a pain block on his left arm. This would give him immediate relief and could last between 3 to 24 hours after surgery. We both looked forward to him receiving any pain relief he could. I kept telling him you just have to hang on a little longer.

3 o'clock came pretty quick and I got up and started to get things ready and packed back in the car. I let Michael sleep until he had to get ready to go. We tried to time his medicine so he could take it about 4 am. That would keep him reasonably comfortable until about 7 am which is when his surgery was scheduled. We left the room and drove to the hospital arriving about 15 minutes before 5 am. As we were driving Michael told me he was nervous. I told him I knew he was but I tried to comfort him and remind him that hopefully it was going to be a wonderful day and finally he could get the pain relief he desperately needed. We both just prayed that the doctor would be able to get the tumor out of his arm with no complications.

We weren't at the hospital waiting area long and they called him back to prep him for surgery. Everyone at this hospital was nice, professional and accommodating. The nurse had Michael change into the proper clothes and she asked him if he was cold. Of course he said he was. The nurse laid a paper type blanket over him and hooked it up to a loud vacuum which blew warm air into the blanket chambers. We had never seen anything like this but after he got used to it he really liked it. If it got too warm they could cool it down. I was just thankful that they were concerned about his comfort. Anytime any nurse, doctor, or any staff member was concerned about his comfort I always felt better. I did not like him to be treated poorly or mistreated at all.

About 6 am our daughters Christie and Eden walked in the room to spend some time with him before he went to surgery. Michael of course was cracking jokes and trying to keep everyone's spirit up. Everyone there was working on keeping his spirit up as well. Right after the girls got there my parents showed up. Mom and dad would not miss this at all. It was amazing that they drove to Oklahoma City that early. It was a couple of hours drive so they really had to get up early to make it.

Eventually Michael's doctor who was to perform the surgery came in the room to mark on Michaels arm, drawing what he was doing to it. Michael just started joking with the doctor. He would say "now doc I hope you have had plenty of coffee this morning." Everyone laughed and then the doctor said he was ready to spend what time it took to get this tumor out of his arm. As soon as his doctor left the room things started moving real quick. The anesthesiologist doctor came into the room and told us he will be administering the pain block in the vein in his neck area and also the anesthesia during the surgery. He asked us to wait outside the room while he gave Michael the pain block. The nurse brought all 5 of us a chair so we could sit while we waited.

The anesthesiologist had walked in the room with tubes of medicine to help block or numb his left arm. It wasn't a minute or two and the doctor walked out and as he walked by he told us I need more medicine his tolerance is very high and we are not there yet. As he came out the door we could get a glance of Michael in his bed. The doctor went back in again with more syringes and then it wasn't long before he came back out for more medicine. The doctor told me I am trying to get him where he needs to be without taking him too far to bring him back. I was in total agreement with that but as much as he was appearing to use made me very nervous. Finally they came out and said that they were successful and we could go in and give him a hug and kiss because they were fixing to take him now to surgery. The doctor told me he is out of it and has a glazed stare but he is ok. We went in one by one and told him we loved him. When I went in he moved his head toward me as I kissed him and I knew he heard me tell him that I loved him. My dad was adamant that we were not leaving that hall until they wheeled him by us on the way to surgery. He was not leaving Michael until he was taken to the surgery room. We waited a few more minutes and then here they came to take him to surgery. The medicine was really taking its toll on him by then and he didn't even notice us. That concerned me but I had to have confidence in all of these doctors. As he was rolled by us we all told him we loved him and would see him right after the surgery.

Mom, Dad, Christie, Eden and I went down to the cafeteria for some breakfast. We were down there an hour or so and the anesthesiologist came down to get himself a bite to eat. He came over to me to let me know that one of his partners was with Michael monitoring him and the doctor has his arm opened and is working on taking the tumor out. I appreciated his update. After that we all went up to the waiting area to wait for any updates from the staff. Every hour or so one of the nurses would update the front desk about Michaels' condition. They in turn would update me. Finally about 3 ½ hours after surgery started his doctor came out to tell me how the surgery went. I was as nervous as I could be. I had received plenty of disappointing news over the past year and I just didn't want this to be one of those days.

The doctor began to tell me most importantly he was able to remove most of the tumor. He told me he didn't think at first he could achieve it. The tumor was wrapped all around his bone, around two nerves and in the muscle. He had to remove one to two inches of Michaels' muscle. The doctor was unable to get the entire tumor out and some smaller microscopic pieces were probably left behind but he told me the radiation will take care of them. He also wanted to tell me that when he took the tumor down to the pathology department that it is from esophagus cancer. That wasn't good news because when the same cancer goes to a second place that places you at stage 4 cancer. This is what they call metastasized. I didn't know what that would eventually really mean but I knew we were up for the battle and at this moment I was just thankful he was able to remove most of that tumor. That was the goal for today.

I went back to the rest of the family and told them the good news. We were all just breathing a sigh of relief and just happy for Michael. As I thought about what the doctor said while I sat there on the sofa with my family I just broke down in tears. The emotion was too much to keep back. I was uncontrollably thankful that the doctor was able to remove the tumor. All I could think was that Michael could finally be out of pain. My daughter came over and held me and I just cried and cried. Not hysterically but tears just rolled down my cheeks and I could not control them or stop them. I was crying but it was a very happy moment and I was so thankful I just couldn't contain it. I was also thankful because I knew Michael had been put through so much. I was just hoping we could start to get past the pain he had to endure and he could begin to get healthy again.

We waited about an hour or so and then a nurse came out to get me so I could see him. He was back from recovery. I went into the room where he was and he was very agitated and angry. The nurse said that one of the drugs they gave him makes some people angry. It took a few minutes but he settled down and everyone was able to come in to see him and tell him they loved him. Then everyone else but me went home because they all have many miles to drive and when Michael was discharged we were going back to the hotel.

For a couple of hours Michaels' oxygen level was really low. After a while I asked the nurse are you sure they are going to discharge him because I am not very comfortable about it. The nurse wasn't either and after talking to the doctor she told me they could keep him overnight for observation. I told her can you please keep an eye on him while I go get a few things from our hotel and I will just stay with him in the room. She promised she would and I left to drive and get what little stuff I left behind. Right before I got to the hotel the nurse called me to tell me he is doing well enough to be discharged now and his oxygen is good even with him asleep. We can discharge him if you want or he can stay in the hospital. I told her please go ahead and get his discharge papers ready. I am on my way back. I knew he would prefer to be out of the hospital if at all possible.

I got back to the hospital and helped him get his clothes on and the nurse had all the discharge papers ready and any items that she felt I would need over the next few days. She wheeled him to my car out front of the hospital and I drove us to the hotel room.

The pain block was still working so his arm was numb. This was good in one respect but also the numb feeling was bothering him and he kept trying to move it. I would tell him to stop and leave it alone. He told me the wrap is hurting him he thought it was too tight. I told him let me loosen it just a little bit and so I did and it helped him feel a little better. I made him as comfortable as I could and finally he fell back to sleep. I watched him sleep and thought to myself I hope and pray that when he wakes up he will feel better. I hope that the tremendous pain that he had been dealing with would finally be over. I figured that the surgery would cause him some pain and discomfort but I also thought that every day he would get better and better.

That night was rough. He was uncomfortable and distressed at times but with his pain medicine and ice packs we got through the night. The next morning he was hurting but I think he was better than the night before. This change gave me confidence. I packed our stuff and loaded the car for the drive back home.

The night before surgery Michael had mentioned to me a Cherokee Trading Post that he would like to visit that was about 20 miles out of our way home but I thought it might be nice to take him there. He didn't feel very excited about going that morning but I told him you are just going to ride and we are going to check it out. It might be fun. When we got there I went around to his door and helped him out of the car. As we walked in the store and slowly walked along looking at all the really neat stuff I could see his mood shifting. We enjoyed walking around and looking at all the neat stuff in the store. We even bought us both a pair of soft moccasins to wear for house shoes at home. They were so comfortable. Later as we left to drive home Michael told me how glad he was that we had visited the store. I knew he would enjoy it and sometimes although time seems real tough you just need to spend a couple of minutes or hours doing something new and fun. It will take your mind off your trouble for just a few minutes or hours whatever the case may be.

We went home to wait for two weeks until Michael could get the stitches out and he could start the radiation treatment. Each day he seemed to get better and the pain would get less and less. We followed the doctors' instructions about the dressing and it appeared that it was healing really well.

What was a welcome sight was that Michael could move his fingers in his hand and within a few days he started moving his elbow and his arm. Within a week or so he was moving it around great. I was very happy about that. At the two week mark we drove to Oklahoma City to have the doctor take out his stitches.

When we saw the doctor who had performed the surgery and his assistant and another doctor who had seen Michael a couple of weeks ago they could not believe their eyes. They told Michael you look like a completely different person. You are energetic, happy and he was moving his arm. This was welcome news to all of them. They told us it was a rough surgery but they are thrilled that it appeared to work out so great. The next step was completing the radiation treatments on his arm. We thanked everyone there and told them how wonderful they were as well. We had just been blessed with the best doctors we could get and believe me we realized that and appreciated it. We wanted them to know how very much we appreciated their work. They thanked us and we started back home.

Chapter Fourteen

When Michaels' chemo and proton doctor received the results of the biopsy they both called me to discuss the best way to move forward. The proton doctor told me that he could recommend two doctors in Tulsa that we could choose from. I told him we trusted his judgment that we would prefer he make the choice for us. He told me that it was great that the tumor was removed and he was confident that the radiation would take care of the residual cancer cells.

The next day the chemo doctor called me to discuss the results as well. As he talked to me about the options he told me, I am just thinking out loud but I do not want to put Michael through more chemo right now. That is a tool we can keep in our tool box. He told me since the PET scan showed cancer only in his arm and because the tumor had been removed and we were going to have radiation on his arm he felt that he could handle the cancer in his arm. He told me when the GI doctor does the next endoscope and if he gets his esophagus open and if anything looks suspicious we will discuss chemo at that time. If there is nothing that looks suspicious then we will not need to do any chemo. The next PET scan was scheduled on June 8, 2015 and we could wait to see what the results of it were. If it was clear he did not want to use chemo. If it showed any other cancer cells then we would cross that challenge at that time.

I told him I agreed 100% I felt getting Michael through the radiation treatments and getting his esophagus open so he could become stronger were the most important items at this time. Then if he needed to endure anything else he would be stronger and healthier. I told the doctor that I was fully aware that we would have to monitor his condition to stay ahead or on top of any cancer that could possibly pop up. But I was extremely impressed and happy that this doctor was so concerned about Michaels' health and was going to proceed cautiously in an effort to help him be able to survive this monster. We were blessed that we had been able to find the absolute best doctors, Thank God!

We were contacted by the radiology doctors' office to set up an appointment to work up a treatment plan for Michaels arm. We went to the appointment and were impressed with this doctor as well. He was confident that he could get rid of the cancer cells in his arm. He felt it would take between 10-15 treatments depending on the original MRI that the surgeon had and a new CAT scan that they would need to perform in the next several days. He told Michael that this type of radiation would be nothing like he had been through with his esophagus since it would be on his arm and no vital organs would be affected. The only type of possible reaction could be sunburn on the skin where the radiation affected. We had been through that so compared to what Michael had endured before we felt this would be much easier.

The doctor office scheduled a CAT scan to make the mold necessary for the radiation treatments. The technicians also marked Michaels' skin for positioning and told him not to remove these marks. He was told it would take about 10 days or so to make the mold and then he would be scheduled for his radiation treatments.

His arm had started to hurt again probably because of the residual cancer cells and also because he hasn't used his arm in months. I thought maybe it was his actual muscles hurting since they had been dormant for so long. One thing was for sure as soon as the radiation treatments would pass the 2nd or 3rd treatment his pain from any cancer cells would be significantly diminished.

The days waiting to start the radiation treatment started to weigh on Michael. He was concerned that each day the cancer would have a better opportunity to spread. Finally 13 days after the visit to the radiation doctor for the measurements for the mold we got the call that they had scheduled the radiation treatments to start the next day. This was great news. Now we could begin to get rid of any residual cancer that was left in his arm. I also was looking forward to the second day or so of radiation to see if the remaining pain that Michael was dealing with would start to diminish. It would be a very welcome day when he could be pain free.

Although it seemed we were close to some resolution Michael started getting more depressed. The radiation doctor didn't think that the regular radiation would cause him as much pain or unpleasantness as he had endured with the proton radiation treatments because there weren't any real vital organs in his arm. Michael was still nervous about it. I can understand that after what he had already been through and of course fear of the unknown is a powerful force. Michael was also depressed because within 5 days he would be at the critical day for the potential of the GI doctor to finally open his esophagus. He had been so disappointed before many times that I believe he just could not believe that it would be possible that he would be able to eat. He was also concerned as I have stated before that putting him under anesthesia gives him so much anxiety on a good day. But now he felt he was even weaker than he ever was before and I believe this was weighing heavy on his heart. He told me I just think it's going to take a lot for them to knock me out for surgery and I just hope they can bring me back. This probably caused him to worry compared to what had happened not long ago during his actual surgery for his arm.

I just had to keep trying to console his fears and remind him how wonderful it was that he could start the radiation tomorrow and we were 5 days away from possibly opening up his esophagus. I kept telling him I love him. He would tell me over and over that he couldn't understand how I could love him since he had lost all the weight and he wasn't what he called "the man he used to be". He said he sees how he looks in the mirror and that he hates how he looks. I told him that is ridiculous! He is my best friend and I love him more than anything. I don't care about any of that. The most important thing to me is that he is around. It just broke my heart to see him so sad. I just had to pray that the radiation went well and that the

GI doctor could open up his esophagus. Many people we know have been praying for us. Each day someone would tell me how they had us in their prayers. I would always tell them "that is what is going to make the difference absolutely." I would always thank them because the power of prayer in my mind is what will give us the edge we need.

Chapter Fifteen

Finally the day came for the endoscope. We looked forward to Michael being able to eat. But honestly I know we were both nervous. I kept thinking about the many times that we had received bad news during these procedures. I just prayed this time would be different. We had to get radiation treatment the same day so we had to be at the hospital early about 7 am. Michael received his radiation treatment then met with his radiation doctor as he did every week. Then we left to go to check in for his endoscope.

We went through the same steps as before, they would take Michael back and prepare him for the procedure but this time we requested the doctor come in to see us before they took him back. When the doctor came in we told him how much we hoped that this time the procedure was successful. What disturbed both me and Michael was the doctor's body language. He shifted back and forth and didn't say anything positive about

Michaels chances just mumbled and said we need to get this going. I felt right then and later Michael told me he felt the same way that this may not go very well. We didn't have much confidence in his demeanor.

Michael told me later that while he waited in the procedure room and they were getting ready to knock him out that the doctor came in and stated let's hurry and get this done I have 6 more to do. Michael wanted to get up and leave then but the thought that possibly it could be successful just kept him laying there. I waited anxiously in the waiting room. Hoping that it would take a long time which I figured meant that the doctor was successful. It didn't take as long as I had hoped for and there stood the doctor again motioning for me to come back to talk to him. As I walked back to a room for him to tell me how it went I noticed how everyone in the room left the room to just me and the doctor.

I immediately said how did it go? The doctor told me it was not good. He then backed up to the wall and said you are going to have to get another doctor that is more aggressive to be successful. He had tried to use the smallest possible tool and it started bleeding and he just didn't feel he was confident enough to be successful. I ask him what does that mean, do I need to look for someone qualified to open his esophagus and where do I look? He told me he could refer us to a couple of doctors but he didn't know if they would take his case. I thought that was curious. Why wouldn't they take his case? I had already told myself if this doctor was not able to be successful after 3 times and making us wait all this time I knew that we were definitely going to find another doctor. I was not expecting however this change in his demeanor and attitude about opening Michaels esophagus. This isn't what he had said the last several times. I was absolutely pissed off and felt about how I did when we first found out Michael had cancer, I was lost and wondering where to turn and who to call for help.

I went back to wait to see Michael in the waiting room. When they called me back to his room it didn't take long and here they came with Michael in a wheelchair. This time he was wide awake and the look on his face said it all. He was pissed as well and ready to get out of there. He asked the nurse to take the IV out of my arm so I could leave. She told him she needed to take his vitals twice and then he could leave. She took his vitals once and told us she would go get his papers for release. After she left Michael turned to me and told me what the doctor said when he came in the room before the procedure. He didn't feel the doctor wanted to take the time necessary to do the job. He was also angry that after multiple times he asked the doctor about what had happened during the procedure the doctor just kept telling him you need to ask your wife. I was shocked, really asking his wife! Why couldn't the doctor tell Michael who was his patient what he had told me? Why did he tell Michael to ask your wife. Was he too busy to even talk to him? What an absolute jerk. This was an unbelievable turn of events that we did not expect. I told Michael what the doctor told me and I kept reminding him we will find the right doctors who will be successful so please keep focusing on that.

The nurse came in with the release papers, took Michaels vitals and removed the IV. I left to get the car and by the time I got to the front door they were waiting for me. Michael got in the car and both of us discussed the events of the day. We were both so pissed off. Michael was depressed and pissed. He had absolutely felt that he would be able to eat. It was a very sad day and my heart just broke for him.

The same day I called the GI doctor's office to see who the doctors were where they sent the referrals. I immediately called that doctors office and talked to a lady that was glad I called. She told me that the doctor had faxed some info on Michael but did not put on the fax what he was requesting or how to contact Michael. I told her some history on Michael and what our goals were, to get his esophagus open. She told me that she would call the GI doctor office to get more info and that she would talk to the doctor. This was a Thursday and she told me the doctor would be out of town through next Wednesday and his normal nurse would be available next Monday. She gave me all the necessary phone numbers that I could use if I needed them.

I called both Michaels proton therapy and chemotherapy doctors and left messages for them to call us back. I hoped maybe they could intervene and help persuade this new doctor to take Michaels case. Then we received a call from the GI doctor office and they told us that the doctor had refused to take Michael's case because he now had metastasized cancer. Again we were shocked. I just believed the doctor had now screwed this up. I just started looking for other doctors who had been successful in what we needed them to do. I also waited for Michael's other doctors to call hoping they would know someone else as well.

First we heard from the proton therapy nurse and she told us that the proton doctor didn't feel comfortable making a call on Michael's behalf. This was pretty disappointing but what could I do? Then his chemotherapy doctor called me. This doctor wanted to know my version of the events. I told him about the procedure, the referrals and how Michael was suffering 20 times or more a day from vomiting the volume of stuff that secreted down is esophagus. He asked me what would you like me to do. I told him I would like you to call this doctor to explain Michaels case and see if he could at least make an appointment to see him. This doctor told me I feel like that the referral doctor hasn't even seen the file or if he has sometimes things look differently on paper and sometimes a doctor to doctor call makes a difference. I was glad to hear this. He went on to tell me he knew a doctor in Oklahoma City that put in stents but he wasn't a fan of stents. He also wanted me to understand that Michael may never be able to have his esophagus open. This is the first time we had heard that possibility. I told him I understand all things possible but I believe we haven't exhausted all our options yet. He agreed and understood my feelings. He told me he would call the referral doctors assistant on Monday and get the doctors cell phone and call him while he was out of town. I was overwhelmed about him doing that. He guaranteed me that he was putting talking to this doctor on his schedule for next week and he would call me as soon as he talked to him. I thanked him for all his help and I hung up the phone thinking to myself what more could I possibly ask for. I felt pretty confident that he could make a difference.

We waited anxiously during the next week expecting a phone call from the chemotherapy doctor at any moment. Finally after several days the phone call came in. He started to tell me that although he tried his best this referral doctor would not take Michaels case and after the discussion with him he could understand why. He went on to tell me that the concern was after all Michael had gone through to this point, arm surgery, radiation in the last month and the fact that the cancer has went to another site even though it's in his arm the doctor was concerned of the toll it would take on Michael especially if his esophagus was perforated during the procedure. The referral doctor refused to take the case for those reasons. The chemo doctor told me I think we need to wait until the PET scan before we put Michael through anything else. If the PET scan is clear then we may have more options. We will discuss that at our visit after the PET scan.

I was very disappointed that the referral doctor would not take the case. I immediately had to figure out how to spin this conversation so Michael would keep positive and keep the faith. I knew we would figure this out and I knew we would be successful. I just didn't know how. I just looked at all the times that we had been told the absolute worst case scenario and he kept beating the odds. I reminded Michael of this and how this was not going to be any different. He absolutely needed to stay strong and determined.

Michael asked me how the doctors think that living like this is living? Throwing up the times he does per day, never eating food again. What if they had to live that way? He believed that they would do anything they could to find someone to open their esophagus. I agreed wholeheartedly.

The chemotherapy doctor called in a patch that would go behind Michael's ear that could help the secretions that plagued Michael's esophagus. The patch was unsuccessful so he removed it. It caused him to get so violently sick the night before his last radiation treatment for his arm that we had to cancel and reschedule that treatment for the next day. On the last treatment Michael endured the treatment but during the doctor visit they could tell he was miserable. He had lost 3 pounds in 2 days because he was sick and unable to eat. The doctor thought that Michael needed fluids and steroids but Michael just wanted to go home. He told us I just can't go through it. You could tell he was weak and sick and tired of being sick and tired. I had been giving him lots of Pedialyte so the doctor thought that would help him as well. The radiation doctor also prescribed another anxiety medicine that also helped nausea so we immediately went to have it filled. The doctor also told me I could use Gatorade because it was cheaper but I preferred using Pedialyte. Each day Michael got stronger and the nausea got better. We added Benadryl which we had used before and it helped dry up some of his drainage.

It did appear although this radiation was supposed to be not a big deal it did take a toll on Michael. I believe that radiation, any kind, has its side effects. I think all kinds make the person tired, sick and burned in some way. To what degree depends on each individual person. Michael had been through a lot and I believe this was tougher on him than most of his doctors thought. This could also be the reason that the referral doctor decided to not take his case especially at this time. Maybe this was a blessing in disguise. I had to believe that. I had to believe God was protecting him and that everything would happen in due time. I knew that his esophagus would get open in due time and when he was stronger to handle it.

During the next couple of weeks I sent out a red alert email to all our children requesting their help in any way possible to network to find a doctor that specializes in what Michael needed. Our oldest daughter immediately went to the internet researching just as I had been doing and she had found a possible option in North Carolina. Our son had contacted a friend of his in the medical field and he called me to tell me he would be working diligently on finding a doctor to help. He told me he would keep in touch and to keep the faith. Our son told me, Mom, this friend of his is even calling France and he knows how important this is and he will keep in touch with you. I went to Joel Olsteens prayer request page and placed a prayer request for God's help to find the right doctor to open Michael's esophagus. I believed that in God's timing we will find the right doctor.

I told Michael that his mission was to get stronger every day, to keep eating as much as he could through his feeding tube so he has gained more weight when we see the chemotherapy doctor after his PET scan. Of course the most important was getting a PET scan. This meant monitoring his ph levels. During the cancer bout in Michael's arm his ph dropped to a 6.0. At this time his ph was 7.0-7.5 generally. A couple of times it dropped to 6.75. We started back on the black strap to make sure that we kept his ph up to a minimum of 7.5 to 8.0. Michael wanted to keep it at 8.0 to make sure we were killing any possible cancer in his body. We monitored and kept it up throughout the next several weeks looking forward to the PET scan. Now I say we were looking forward to the PET scan and that is not actually a true statement. What I mean is we are nervous and anxious as everyone is when they are going to get this test taken. But we were looking forward to seeing if the PET scan was clear what our possibilities would be at that time for opening his esophagus open.

Chapter Sixteen

The day came for the next PET scan and although we were nervous I think this time we were more optimistic than before. We had believed that since the last one only showed cancer in Michael's arm and he had surgery and radiation to deal with that issue, we really were cautiously confident that this time we were cancer free. My parents had made the trip as they had many times for support, and as before we waited for Michael to have the test. This time the test was taking longer than before so I went to the desk to see what was going on. They told me that he was getting dressed and would be out shortly.

When Michael came out to the lobby he looked pretty frayed. I asked what had happened and he began to tell us that they had to repeat the test because the first one he was unable to complete. They had put him into the chamber or the coffin as he likes to refer to it, they had strapped him down so he could not move and they had turned the microphone off so they could not hear him. Because his esophagus is closed the natural secretions in your esophagus began to fill up his esophagus and he was feeling as though he was drowning. He was yelling for the staff but they could not hear him. They must have seen his feet or something because they came back in the room and heard him yell. They had to pull him out so he could throw up and he was having real anxiety. Making things worse because they had to stop the test and it needed to be repeated. After he settled down they were able to repeat the test but this time they kept the microphone on.

As he told us the story we knew that had to be scary and we thanked God he hadn't drowned in there. I couldn't believe they weren't watching him. Our next appointment was with the doctor who would give us the results of the PET scan. Michael was focused on working with this doctor to be his advocate with an appropriate experienced doctor who could open his esophagus up. He had endured so much pain, treatment and disappointment that today we were finally hoping for some good news.

We left Mom and Dad in the waiting room as we went back to talk to the doctor. Michael had lost more weight which wasn't good but he had been through surgery and radiation and 3 endoscopes since the last PET scan so he thought that is probably normal.

The doctor walked into the room and Michael was so glad to see him. Michael asked the doctor what options are available to get his esophagus open so he can eat. His doctor said let's talk about that in a few minutes, first let's talk about the PET scan. We both took a breath and thought, oh that doesn't sound good. Michael then asked him what the results of the PET scan were.

His doctor started to tell us the cancer is back in the esophagus and now it is affecting both of his adrenal glands. We sat in silence and then Michael asked well how do we fix it? The doctor looked at him and said we can't. You have 2 months to live. 4 months with chemotherapy treatment but before we consider if you are a candidate for chemotherapy I will need to ask you a series of questions.

The questions included how much during the day is he awake, does he stay in bed all day or is he active and if so how much and so on. Michael could tell what he was looking for and at times I think he answered the questions based on what the doctor needed to hear so he could get the treatment not necessarily what the facts were.

This was Michael's call as far as I was concerned and I agreed with him that he needed to try to beat it with all tools at his disposal. As Michael instructed the doctor that he wanted to fight this battle the doctor looked at me for my opinion and I agreed with Michael let's see how it goes and how he tolerates the treatment.   The doctor agreed to schedule the treatment and told us it would begin the following week.

The doctor also informed us that generally the chemotherapy treatment calls for a combination of three chemo drugs but because of Michael's health we would start out with just one and see how he tolerated it. The doctor also told us he wouldn't even give his mother the three drugs together. We were confident in this doctor and knew he was calculating Michael's health into the chemotherapy treatment he would schedule for him. I was aware there would also be premedication as before and any other drugs necessary to help make it through this treatment. The one difference this time was Michael would need to have the port placed in his heart that he had dreaded. Because of the chemo treatment before his veins in his arms had suffered enough so this was the best way to proceed.

Finally the doctor told Michael about a GI doctor that he had discussed Michael's case with and discussed if he would consider taking it to try to open his esophagus. We were given his name and told to make an appointment.

As anyone can imagine as we left the doctors' office we were in shock. Inside I was terribly emotional. Mom and dad waited for the news and could tell it wasn't good. In the hallway outside the doctors' office we shared what the doctor said. Mom said "Oh my God, this is so unfair." They were both sad and shocked.

I told them the plan and that we intended to fight. Michael told them he had received so many death sentences in the last year and a half, what is one more. We gave each other hugs and kisses and drove home.

I was devastated but determined to research what else we could do. The doctor had told us if we would like to look at someone else he wouldn't have his feelings hurt but we insisted that we have confidence in his ability. I did however go back to research. I kept reminding Michael that the doctor can only go by statistics that they have and that people are exceptions to those statistics all the time. So far he had been beating the statistical odds and I expected that he would continue to do so.

I immediately made the appointment for later this same week to have the port placed so chemo could begin the following week. Although Michael was so weak he went through the port placement surgery with flying colors and was released to go home outpatient. I was happy how well things went.

The following week we showed up for the lab, the doctor appointment and finally the chemotherapy infusion. This time Michael would have the pre-medications and what they call a chemo push which is a small version of the chemotherapy that was ordered and after that was given then a small bag with a pump that would deliver chemotherapy at a slower rate was placed on Michael that we would need to wear for 46 hours and then come back to the infusion center to have it removed. This treatment would access the port in his heart so Michael would not need to have any other sticks for blood or chemo. This part he was happy about. This bag was weird for him to get used to but he tolerated it and for the next two days we were very careful where this bag was concerned.

Because Michael was having so much problem with secretions and throwing up constantly and it was taking a toll on him he asked me to please make an appointment with the GI doctor that the chemo doctor had referred us to. Within days we had an appointment and we drove back to

Oklahoma City to meet this doctor and see what if anything could be done to open his esophagus.

The doctor was in surgery we were told but the head nurse told us the game plan and the complications that could occur from trying to open the esophagus to put a stent in. These included perforation which would require opening Michael's chest up and doing a major surgery to close the perforation if that occurred. We had explained that with the chemo treatment it was possible the cancer would shrink and maybe he would have an easier job to open the esophagus if we waited to see if the treatment worked. The nurse told us the chemo doctor had told them that he wasn't confident that the treatment would work at all. That statement concerned me. I must say I still don't believe that the chemo doctor ever said that at all. He may have said that the statistics aren't optimistic but I don't believe he said it the way she told us. Michael told the nurse let us think about it. You could tell they wanted to schedule this procedure immediately and that gave us both great pause.

On the drive home for the first time since we learned Michael had this type of cancer he said I can just keep using this feeding tube. He was not in a hurry to possibly get cut open as the nurse had described and he believed that if that happened he would not probably survive that type of surgery. We both agreed let's wait and see about how he does during the treatment.

Maybe the tumor would shrink. We had faith and that's the decision that was made. I was extremely proud of him making that decision the way he did.

Chapter Seventeen

The following week was the next chemotherapy treatment scheduled. Before each treatment lab would be drawn to check Michael's health and then we would have a doctor appointment. At this appointment we are told Michael's lab shows he is good to go as far as his chemotherapy treatment today. Then the doctor paused and told us I have some news. My heart sank, what kind of news could he have?

He began to tell us that after our last appointment he contacted the entity that had Michael's original biopsy material from the year before and had it tested for the HER2 gene. He proceeded to tell us that the test showed that Michael's test was positive for the HER2 gene. Only 20% of esophageal cancer patients test positive for this gene. For those that test positive there is a targeted therapy called Herceptin that has been approved by the FDA for these patients. This gene can also be found in some breast cancer patients and this drug can help them as well. I thought this was fantastic news. I had been praying for a miracle and I believed that this was our answer.

I also was impressed that the doctor decided to have his biopsy checked. I believed it was from our demeanor and conversation the appointment before he could tell we were all in for this fight. We trusted him and I think he went back to the drawing board to see what else if anything he could try or do to help on his end.

He told us that Michael would have to have a test to check his heart and if that looked good that on the next treatment he would add the targeted therapy to his treatment plan. I was very excited.

We continued to the infusion center to receive the scheduled chemotherapy treatment. When we came back in two days to have the chemotherapy bag removed the doctor had scheduled the electrocardiogram to check Michaels' heart. I was pretty confident about this test because he had several EKG's over the last several months and every one of them had checked out good. It was amazing what he had been enduring and how strong his heart was through it all.

During the electrocardiogram Michael asked the nurse taking the test how things looked. She told him look at this part of your heart, which he could see on a screen. She began to tell him how strong this part of his heart was and that over her many years working there that he was the second best heart she had ever seen. That was welcomed news. That meant he would be able to receive the targeted therapy.

The doctor told us that he wanted Michael to receive four chemotherapy treatments with targeted therapy before his next PET scan would be scheduled. I was in agreement with that. The next PET scan would determine if the targeted therapy treatment was working.

Because Michael had been so sick to his stomach so much it would cause him to become dehydrated. On his next doctor visit we were also told he had low sodium levels and his hemoglobin was low. He also was experiencing a bad cough. We didn't know if the episode during the PET scan caused him to aspirate but Michael was also getting pneumonia. On top of everything else his immunity was low due to the chemotherapy. This meant on top of fighting cancer we were going to have to battle multiple challenges at the same time.

For low sodium Michael would receive extra fluids during treatment and I was told to add 2 crushed sodium chloride tablets a day to his formula. I also started giving him Pedialyte instead of water with his formula and medicine. For his hemoglobin the doctor added a specific shot for 2 treatments until his hemoglobin reached acceptable levels.

Amazingly, at one point Michael's blood pressure was 84/44 but he still endured his treatment. He was confused and not really with it which is also a sign of low sodium. We had so many challenges so we would have to prioritize which ones were more important. Low sodium at this time was the priority. As soon as we got his sodium closer to normal the more normal he became. He would become more alert and appeared like he was back to his old self. Monitoring his demeanor became necessary for me to be able to tell how well we were keeping his sodium levels close to normal.

Just about the time we are winning the sodium battle his vitals showed his oxygen level in the 80's. This is not an acceptable level. Under 90 you need oxygen. The doctor monitored him for a while during treatment to see if going under 90 was a fluke or something more serious. Unfortunately he was having a problem keeping his oxygen levels up to normal so the doctor put an order in for oxygen around the clock. The order was placed while we were at the doctors' office in Oklahoma City and by the time we had traveled back home the company was ready to deliver the oxygen to our home. I could not believe how fast they were but I was very thankful. We probably would have ended up in the emergency room again that night if we had not received the oxygen in such a timely manner.

Again during this time frame Michael aspirated and this created pneumonia. Day by day as we struggled to get his sodium levels normal he seemed to slip further and further away. One evening it was as if he was drowning while he slept. I went downstairs and wrestled with what to do.

I told my daughter I don't know whether to take him to the hospital or not. I know he wouldn't want to die at the hospital and I knew he would prefer to die at home but I just don't know what to do. My daughter told me, "Mom, you have to do what you can live with." That was absolutely right. So I went back up to the room and although I had asked Michael many times before let's go to the doctor and he would tell me no. This time I told him Michael we really need to go to the doctor and have you checked out. He looked at me and said okay. That was all I needed to get working on getting him dressed and figuring out how to get him downstairs. I had originally thought I may need to call an ambulance but my daughter and I were able to get him to the car.

As soon as I pulled up to the hospital they came to the car with a wheel chair and took him straight back to the urgent care area of the emergency room. I was impressed with their speed of helping him. This gave me encouragement.

The nurses tried to make him comfortable. They put him on oxygen and started an IV. As this process was taking place the doctor came into the room and asked me what was the plan? I was shocked that he would ask me that. I looked at him and said the plan is do whatever it takes to save his life!

I would have to endure that question many times more since Michael was a cancer patient and had esophagus cancer that had metastasized. The impression from some doctors was they just didn't see the purpose to postpone the inevitable. They couldn't understand why we wouldn't just give up and Michael could just go ahead and die. I just felt everyday he is alive is one more precious day we get to spend together. Another conversation, another one of his jokes and another time for him to tell me how much he loved me and for me to give him a kiss and tell him how much I loved him. We were not ready to give up. I could only imagine that a lot of people make different decisions and just let their loved one slip away. I was going to fight to keep Michael alive as long as he was willing to fight to stay alive. I couldn't imagine making any other kind of decision than that.

So with the instructions from me the doctor said okay and things started to happen. They put him on constant antibiotic IV and other medicines and admitted him to the hospital. He was transferred to ICU or Intensive Care.

He spent two days in ICU and then was moved to the Respiratory Care Unit for 3 days. After a grueling 3 days, on the 4th day it was if he woke up and wondered where he was. I could tell the change in him and I told him welcome back. He immediately wanted to go home and by the 5th day the doctor released him with antibiotics to take at home. Amazingly he had beat pneumonia.

The next day when we were home I told him we need to get you cleaned up, give you a shower and wash your hair so you'll feel better. As I began to take off the bandage the hospital had put on his feeding tube I had trouble getting it off. They had put so much tape on there so I got a pair of scissors and I was trying to be very careful but all of a sudden I snipped what I thought was tape and cloth but it was his feeding tube. Oh my god, I had cut off all of his tube but about an inch. Stomach contents started to drain out and I just started to freak out. I told Michael oh my god I can't believe I did that and I grabbed a Q-tip and stuck in the feeding tube hole to stop it from leaking and we used a string to tie the tube shut. What a 911 crisis. Michael was so calm but I was so upset that I had made such a huge mistake. I was so tired from being in the hospital 24/7 with him and I couldn't believe that now we had to turn around and go back to the hospital to have his feeding tube replaced. Without the use of the feeding tube he couldn't receive his food but also all of his medicine he needed every 4 hours. This was a real crisis. I just got everything together and got him ready to go, told the family what happened and that we were on our way back to the hospital. Of course we had to stay overnight because they had to prepare him for surgery the next day. It also meant they could only give him pain medicine through IV and this was not enough to control his pain so until we got the feeding tube fixed he was going to have to endure some unwelcome pain that the nursing staff could not get totally under control.

The next morning they took him down to the interventional radiology department where they can watch by x-ray as they remove and replace his feeding tube. They were able to replace it without knocking him out so that was one part of this unpleasant event that worked out well. With the feeding tube back in place now he could have his normal medicines and we could get his pain under control and go back home so we could get back to business as usual going through cancer treatment or so I thought.

We went home and within a couple of days Michael started to have problems breathing again and told me to run him up the emergency room in Sapulpa. We thought maybe like before they could give him a breathing treatment and a shot and he would feel better. This time would be different. The doctor told us he had nodules on his lungs which mean he's either aspirated again or he has cancer in his lungs. The doctor told us he needs to stay a minimum of seven days to get over pneumonia with IV antibiotics.

Michael was not happy with going back to the hospital especially for 7 days but this time he understood it was necessary and he was amicable with getting it over with.

The Sapulpa hospital was not capable of keeping patients for this type of treatment and length so Michael was transported to the same hospital he was in the last time with pneumonia. It was also nice because they already had all of his previous records. For seven days he stayed in the hospital and for seven days I stayed there 24/7 with him. He just did not want me to leave him at all. As long as I was there he felt safe. And again, after this visit they told him after they took a chest x-ray he had beaten pneumonia again. I was just amazed at how tough he was. But also very thankful and I knew a lot of people were also praying everyday for him. So finally we go back home and I am hoping we are done with hospitals for a while. It had seemed we had almost been living in one.

Now Michael was pretty independent and he was determined to try to walk to and from the bathroom although I would normally have to help him. Eventually we got him a walker to help keep him steady and more stable. But the day after we got home from the hospital, Michael got up while I was asleep and all of a sudden I heard a loud crash. I jumped up and went over to see what happened and Michael fell on the floor by the bathroom and busted his head wide open. It was awful. I picked him up and asked him what happened and he told me he just fell. I of course told him do not ever get out of bed without me knowing it and helping you to and from the bathroom. But this cut in his forehead was bad so back to the emergency we went. Fortunately this time they stitched him up and we were able to come right back home.

After this incident we had to make some adjustments in our program. He had to agree that although he was independent he would make sure he had help to and from wherever he wanted to go whether it was to and from the bathroom or downstairs or on a walk. He would always need someone's help from now on.

Now we could get back to the cancer treatments and the targeted therapy that we were hopeful would make the difference in his recovery.

Chapter Eighteen

After about a month of back and forth to Oklahoma City getting Michael's treatment it was time for a PET scan to see if we were making progress. This was always a nervous time because you always had anxiety about the kind of news you could get and you were also hopeful that finally you would get some good news that the treatment is working.

We had to wait several days for the results and we had just resigned our thinking no matter what the results were we were going to keep on fighting no matter what. When we went in to see the doctor he looked puzzled. He told us I just really don't believe it but the targeted therapy is working. Now I was confused that he was surprised that it was working but I felt that meant that Michael is the exception to the rule. The doctor told us that the cancer in one of his adrenals was almost gone, the other adrenal was significantly smaller and that the same was true with his esophagus. This was fantastic news! When we got up to leave the doctor's office, Michael told the doctor it was all him and thank you so very much. The doctor told him no I believe your wife is what is making the difference. My response was it is a team effort. Then the doctor stopped and told us shaking his head this is "divine intervention." This was the kind of day every one dealing with cancer looks forward to, good news! And that maybe finally something is working and we are going to beat this monster. We went home, called all our family and friends and gave them the good news. We wanted to share some good news with them for a change because we were all tired of all the bad news it seemed we kept getting.

The next day was our 23rd Anniversary so it made that celebration even more special. Dad wanted to take Michael striper fishing so he had scheduled a guide to take Michael, my dad, my brother, our son, and our grandson striper fishing two days after we got this good news. Our grandson was important on the trip on the boat because he was so familiar with giving Michael his medicine and fluids, formula or anything else he should need through his feeding tube.

We went down the night before and spent the night with my parents and we had a wonderful visit. My parents took such good care of both of us but really dotted on Michael. Mom kept him covered with a blanket to keep him warm because with his weight loss he was cold all the time. But everyone looked forward to their fishing trip and hoped they would have a lot of success catching a mess of fish to cook.

Mom and I and my sister in law visited and spent some quality time together while the guys were out on their fishing trip. When they got back we got some pictures of them all together and it was just so special that they could spend this time together.

Michael and I both just really enjoyed it. They didn't get as many fish as they wanted but being together out on the lake with the wind in your hair was such a wonderful thing for Michael. And most important, memories were made and quality time spent. We gave everyone hugs and kisses like always. We told everyone we loved them and we headed back home. The following week it was back to business as usual and more cancer treatments. Looking at the pictures taken from that day it was amazing how frail and weak Michael was and you could tell that by how he looked in the pictures and how he kept losing more and more weight. It was incredible that he was standing, walking with his cane and with help but still pushing himself to go forward. It just gave our entire family the belief that he was one tough guy and that he was going to beat this. We all believed that, prayed about that and more than anything in the world wanted that to be the end result.

We went about another month or so traveling to Oklahoma City for cancer treatments every week. As anyone knows that has ever dealt with Cancer it is devastating on your family and your finances. We were financially in trouble. Our house was in foreclosure, we had borrowed and begged for money throughout a lot of this time to pay Michaels insurance premiums and to pay for gas to and from Oklahoma City and Tulsa and for Pedialyte and other items that I needed to get just to help him with his care not to mention his formula which the insurance company didn't pay for or for my food. I just don't know how we made it as long as we did but finally we were out of resources. The family that would help was unable to because they didn't have the funds and the family and friends that could just decided they wouldn't help anymore. This was a heartbreaking blow, how were we going to be able to pay his insurance to keep him alive! I know people deal with this same question every day and it breaks my heart that anyone has to endure it.

Now during the past couple of years I have worked part time. But the amount of money that I had made was not enough to meet our expenses. Michael was unable to work and I was unable to work more and take care of him. I was his caregiver and if I was gone from him for any length of time Michael would panic.

We sold what we could and we were at a point in our life that we were out of options. I have to impress on everyone this was the most embarrassing, painful, and heartbreaking thing to endure and on top of that we were in a position to have to ask or beg others for help.

Michael called everyone he knew and begged everyone he knew and finally a friend he hadn't spoken to in a while, but an absolute angel from God told us he would get a hold of his church. They have a benevolence fund and maybe they could help with paying his insurance. We were behind one payment and had two days to pay it or the policy cancelled which meant no more cancer treatment. This friend's church pastor called and spoke with Michael and had me send him an invoice from our insurance company. Now it was over $1,600 a month premium. Within a couple of hours the guy from the church called Michael and told him to please tell your wife that we not only paid the past due premium but we paid the current premium as well. We both just broke down and cried. What a blessing from God! There is no way we could ever repay them for the blessing they gave us that day. Nor could we ever begin to put into words how much it meant to us. And unknown to us at the time the church was not done. They rallied behind us like I have never seen before. A couple called and told us they wanted to drive us back and forth to Oklahoma City for Michaels' treatments. They brought me snacks, covered Michael in blankets to keep him warm, prayed with us many times and most importantly became very good friends, the kind that are priceless. They were going through their own cancer battles and yet they were going out of their way to make our life easier. It was just awesome to watch how wonderful God is. Michael loved God with all his heart and so do I but I still was overwhelmed with all the love from so many people who didn't even know us at all.

Chapter Nineteen

It seemed that things were looking up but then I woke up early one morning and looked at Michael and he did not look good. One side of his face was drooping and he was not coming around although he would acknowledge me. I immediately ran down to tell my daughter I have to call an ambulance please go up and stay with him. We were all used to moving at a moments' notice because we were always on alert for anything. I called the ambulance and they came pretty quick. Since we were upstairs they had to call the fire department to help take him downstairs because of how our house was set up. The EMS guy told me it appears that he has had a stroke or he is sepsis. But he tried to reassure me that if we got it in time that he should be okay. I rode in the ambulance with Michael and my daughter notified the family and our other daughter and son and our granddaughter got to the hospital pretty quick behind me. I also notified the friends we had from church. The chaplain from the hospital came in and prayed over Michael and it looked pretty grim. The hospital had run tests on Michael's head to see what was causing the problem he was having. Then the doctor on duty came in and began to tell me what was going on. I motioned for him to go out in the hallway because whatever news it was if it was bad I did not want Michael to hear it even if they thought he was out of it. The doctor told me he was sorry to inform me that he has a mass in his brain that is probably the cancer which has spread. It is unknown at this time if it could be swelling but he was too weak to endure a biopsy or brain surgery so the doctor was going to treat him for swelling and see if they made a difference. He had also aspirated so we were again fighting pneumonia. The doctor asked me if he had a DNR, do not resuscitate. I told the doctor that he does not. He said you need to prepare yourself because we may get to a point where you have to make the decision for him. I told him we were not at that point yet so let's work on getting him better. The doctor admitted him back to Intensive Care. I did not feel comfortable with this doctor and I sent a message to Michael's primary care doctor to let him know my feelings. This doctor seemed more concerned about turning treatment off than with trying to fix him. This really concerned me. I was aware of how grim our situation was but I refused to play God and decide when Michael should die. This was God's decision not mine!

I notified my parents and a couple of Michael's friends. I went back into Michael's room and noticed that both of his pupils were different sizes. The nurse came in and they took him down to an emergency CAT scan of his brain. I don't know what happened when he was gone but when he got back they had him on a special machine pushing oxygen into him to get his oxygen levels up and his respiration was in the 30's. The doctor called me out into the hallway and told me that the discussion we had earlier about whether to put a ventilator in him to help him breathe needed to be decided on now. That I needed to understand that when his respiration got up to 40, his body would start to give out and it would be too late to help him at that time. You can either put him on a ventilator, leave him off a ventilator and I can take him off his medicines and make death even come quicker if you would like. That really pissed me off. I knew that Michael had told me he didn't want to live on life support but still I did not want to make this decision. I told the doctor not to put him on a ventilator but I want him to continue getting any of the medicines he needs to help him be more comfortable including the antibiotics to help him get over the pneumonia. I just started praying for a miracle. My daughter asked how come he hadn't received any breathing treatments so they were ordered as well. With that decision made, the doctor told me it is only a matter of time. So I contacted all our family, friends and our church family. The couple from the church came up and prayed and saw us and met the rest of our family, and our grandchildren sat on the side of his bed and read to him although he would look at them and could only say, ok, yea, or I love you. He was not himself at all. It was hard to watch but we all loved him so much. Everyone was crying, we just couldn't help it, our heart was breaking, we were losing him and we were helpless to stop it. Then he started coughing. Our son said, Dad, cough! Every time he coughed his respiration rate went down. We all had been watching the monitor sometimes in horror but still hoping for the impossible. He had almost got to the magical number of 40 but within an hour or two we were back to 20. Unbelievable! He was again beating the odds. Thank God I didn't put him on a ventilator!

After several hours it appeared he was becoming more stable and most of the family and extended family were able to go home. I of course would stay as always 24/7 by his side. The next day the doctor came in and told me he couldn't believe the turn around. I was really unhappy with this doctor. He had not been giving him any nourishment, we had to request breathing treatments and antibiotics, these all made the difference. That is why I couldn't leave his side. If I left at all, one of our family members would have to be there. And believe me our oldest daughter was one of his staunchest supporters when it came to making sure he was comfortable and getting what he needed.

This hospital stay would be much different than the rest. This doctor did not give him the level of nourishment he needed so within the ten days we were there Michael would lose 20 pounds. He told us you gotta get me out of here, look at me. The doctor wanted to send him to a skilled nursing home but he wanted to go home. He did not want hospice so we were discharged to go home with home health. Home health was something I had just signed up with before this hospital stay but we had not used yet.

The good things that happened during our stay were the many wonderful people from the church whom we hadn't met who came to see us, who sent gift cards, snacks, reading material, blessings and prayers for us throughout the difficult hospital stay. They meant the world to us. Then on the day of Michael's discharge the church pastor came to visit and told us they had paid another insurance premium for us so we don't have to stress out about that. I was just amazed constantly how loving and caring these people are. I just prayed God blessed them all more than they could dream of because of the wonderful things they had done for us. Michael's friend who got us in touch with his church came up multiple times as well as his wife and also bearing gifts and I can't ever thank them enough. Michael told them all himself personally how much he appreciated it and I know they could tell how serious his situation was and how much he loved God and he loved them for their blessings and prayers.

I was glad to be able to take him home. While in the hospital the nurses had to give him bathes and because he had become so weak and immobile he was started on adult Depends. This way it helped eliminate fall risks but it meant I had to move him back and forth and change him. It took at least two nurses to do it and I was going to have to do most of it by myself. I could get some help from my daughter and son in law downstairs, my grandsons or brother but most of the time it would just be me. I just had to reach deep inside and tell myself you are just going to have to get the strength to pull this off. He is counting on you. And that is what I did. The other challenge we had that had happened to him during this hospital stay was that he had contracted herpes virus on his lips, in his mouth, and on his skin and down his throat. The doctor wouldn't give him any medicine for it and it was painful and it was extremely hard on him. As soon as I got him home the home health nurse called another doctor and got him some medicine to help him with this condition.

Chapter Twenty

The next seven days were a battle like no other. He was in incredible pain with the herpes on his face, he was losing his voice, getting weaker, and his body was having a harder time fighting all the battles of all the different things attacking it. Cancer, pneumonia, herpes, low sodium, starvation from not getting the adequate nutrition during his hospital stay, and the embarrassment of being bed ridden living with adult Depends. During his hospital stay he tried to make fun as much as possible calling the nurses and saying, cleanup on aisle 8. We were in room 8 so everyone thought he was quite the joker. And he was but by the time we got home he was fading and I could tell. While in the hospital he kept saying I want to go home to be around our dogs and cats. But when he got home he didn't want them around him. I am not sure why that was but he was really struggling. They wanted to help but they were unable to comfort him this time. It took 24 hours around the clock to deal with everything that was necessary to take care of him after he came home. I was getting sick, I didn't know at the time but I was getting pneumonia as well. About 7 days after we came home from the hospital, it was around 3 o'clock in the morning, time for Michaels' dose of medicine so I began to give it to him in his feeding tube. All of a sudden he started getting really sick, throwing up constantly. The only thing that had changed is the home health had started him on a new antibiotic. I had to keep holding him upright so he could throw up in a bag. Now his esophagus was blocked so I couldn't figure out where all this liquid was coming from. This process started to take a toll on me so Michael told me to call your brother, who was down stairs in case we needed help. I did and he came up stairs. We were both now in a fight to save Michael's life. Michaels' oxygen level started to drop, he was having trouble breathing. I gave him breathing treatments, he would throw up, I would give him oxygen and we would constantly monitor his oxygen. Less than 90 oxygen means he needs oxygen. He dropped to 80 then 70. Respiration started to get really quick, still throwing up, still not able to breathe. I called a home health nurse and she came over. By the time she got there Michael had lost control of all his body fluids which I knew was a sign someone is close to dying. My brother told me the look on my face was frightening when that happened. I knew oh my God, I am losing him. All of a sudden Michael looked up at me and told me, I love you more than anything! I told him I loved him more than anything too and I just grabbed his upper half and cuddled his head and cried. The home health nurse got there and his oxygen was in the 40's. How he was alive was incredible. She asked if I wanted the ambulance called and I did. They got there and gave him a breathing treatment and oxygen. The EMS lady asked me do you want me to call a doctor and do the paperwork or what's the plan? I said you need to talk to him. He can talk to you. She went over to Michael and asked him Michael, can you hear me? He said yes. Michael do you want me to put a tube down your throat so it can help you breathe? He said yes. He confirmed that 6 more times by the time they got him down to the ambulance. After they got him into the ambulance, sedated him and put a tube down to help him breathe, he never was able to speak again. Home health told me it is unbelievable he is still alive, he is not finished with something yet. He is hanging on for something. I knew he didn't want to leave me.

While the EMS personnel were working to get Michael down to the ambulance our animals were going crazy, trying to break down the doors, they desperately wanted to help him, and they could tell he was in real danger.

As we had in the past, the family was notified and everyone showed up at the hospital. The emergency room doctor told me several parts of his body were failing and she was having a problem keeping his oxygen levels up. She worked on him for hours until she could move him to a specific Intensive Care floor and this time he had a really good doctor assigned to his care.

That doctor came to meet me, had me update any information about his care I felt he needed to know since I was his caregiver and he also wanted me to know that do not be surprised in the next 48 hours if you hear a code blue. He is in a seriously critical situation. He had another pulmonary doctor coming to check why they couldn't keep his oxygen up so he would keep me updated.

The pulmonary doctor found that Michael had a hole in his airway that once they got the air tube past that hole they were able to get his oxygen stable. They put him in a sedated state to keep him calm. They told me they thought the cancer had caused a hole in his airway that went also to his stomach which is why he was throwing up all the liquid throughout the night. I didn't know if I believed that or if the EMS had punctured a hole when she ventilated him but my daughter told me, mom, he was having trouble keeping his oxygen up before the EMS got there.

For the next 48 hours we lucked out and we didn't have a code blue. They thought they had Michael sedated but when my daughter was in his room and was talking to him he started to move his arm. He would look at her and follow her around the room. I was in the waiting room so my grandchildren ran to get me and I went in. When you went into his room you had to put on gloves and certain clothing. I went in his room and his eyes were open. I told him I loved him so very much and that I was there and would not leave. He was looking at me and trying to say something because you could see his mouth move around from the ventilator but he couldn't say anything because of the ventilator. The nurse realized that they didn't have him sedated like they were supposed to so they upped the medicine and Michael was put under sedation. After that when they would try to get him to respond he would not respond to any of us.

About 5 days into this stay, many nurses and doctors were trying to get me to prepare to take him off of the ventilator. I just kept faith that he would bounce back like he always had before. About 5 days into this hospital stay the nurse called me in to tell me he was close to A FIB. I needed to understand that when they had to resuscitate him and when they start the compression on his chest, he is so frail it will cause his ribs to break. Our son was in the room and I saw tears in his eyes but he never flinched. He knew I had to make the decision. I told the nurse I do not want that. I do not want you to break his ribs. He's been through enough. Do everything you can with medicine. He told me okay we will put him on a limited DNR. I told him that would be good. Our son turned toward me and told me, I think that's a good decision mom. And again for a couple of days the medicine they gave him appeared to keep him stable.

I had been sleeping on the floor in the waiting room and was getting really sick. I thought if he's stable maybe I better go home one night. I went to check on him and noticed his numbers were not looking good. Oxygen was falling, and the ventilator wasn't helping, heart rate rising, blood pressure erratic. I called our children and told them I thought it looked grim. They all rushed to the hospital. We all stayed in the room with him for several hours, holding his hands, staring at the monitor and then amazingly again it appeared he started to stabilize. Everyone went home around midnight except our oldest daughter. But everyone stayed on alert and told me to call them immediately if there was any change.

It didn't take an hour or so and Michael was back in distress. The nurse on duty told our daughter I hate giving him these medicines they call pressures because eventually it will cause his fingers and toes to fall off. Our daughter came and told me what she had said and I went and confronted her about that statement. I told her I did not want that to happen to him. He was already holding a lot of fluid. His belly, arms and hands were huge. I could tell we were erring on the side of torture. I told the nurse that I did not want him to have any more of that medicine so she called the doctor. The doctor told me then his recommendation was that we needed to go ahead and remove the ventilator. I finally agreed I knew we had reached the point where keeping him alive was torturing him. But taking him off the ventilator really scared me. I did not want to see him gasp for air and I wanted him to have the most peaceful transition when he got to that point.

Our son went directly into the waiting room, he was very emotional and told me he could not be in the room during that part, he was just too upset. Our other daughter left the room thinking she had time to go to the restroom. We were told it would take the respiration unit some time to get down to his room to remove the ventilator. Our oldest daughter and I stayed in the room with Michael. I held one hand on one side and she on the other holding his other hand. Both of us just kept staring at the monitor at the same time I kept feeling the weight of this terrible decision I just had to make. Knowing that the man I love, the absolute love of my life is close to the end of his life, I am going to lose him and he will soon know the mystery of life and death.

They had just upped his pain medicine before I made this decision and all of a sudden we could hear him start to snore. We thought that was great, finally they have made him comfortable. His blood pressure was 56/34. I thought to myself that is so low but his heart is so strong. His heart rate was 100. Then the nurse came in to take away some of the fluids that had been hooked up to him and all of a sudden Michaels heart rate went from 100 to 30, then 29, 28, 27, 26, 25, 24, 23, 22, 21, 20, 19, 18. 17, 16, 15, 14, 13, 12, 11, 10, 9, 8, 7, 6, 5, 4, 3, 2, 1, 0 ----------------------. As soon as his heart rate went from 100 to 30 the nurse said, "oh my god he's going to go on his own." The ventilator was still in. My daughter and I watched in horror as his heart rate went to 0 and then flat lined. As we cried she told me, "Mom, dad did not want you to live with making that decision so he went on his own." Others told me he had waited until he knew I was ready for him to go.

Believe me, and many people witnessed it throughout the last 21 months that I was never ready for him to leave me. I did realize what was happening to him and what he must have been going through had to be torture. In the end God decided the moment that Michaels' life was to end. I thank God for that. And I absolutely believe that Michael is out of pain and he is in a much better place.

Our daughter that wasn't in the room was upset she wasn't there when he passed; she thought we had more time. Our son was truly upset as were all our family and friends. My brother, our children and their spouses came up to the hospital for support. I can only say that it was a blur for me. It felt like my heart stopped as well. I felt guilty because I couldn't save his life, and heartbroken that my best friend in the whole world was gone.

I left the hospital in shock. I insisted on driving myself and I knew I needed to go to the doctor and get me some medicine because I was sick.

When I got there the doctor was very concerned for me, because I was visibly upset and when he found out I had just lost my husband he understood why. He told me I had pneumonia and he gave me a shot and medicine to help me get better. I had been so run down taking care of him that it took me several months to get over the pneumonia.

While I had been in the hospital I had researched what happens after someone dies in the hospital and it told how your arrangements need to be made and if you cremate someone you need to have the family come to the hospital before the funeral home comes to pick them up or you won't be able to see them. That's not what happened but I did realize I better get these arrangements in order just in case. I had left the hospital about a day before he died long enough to meet with a funeral home to make some arrangements. Our oldest daughter had taken charge of most of the arrangements but I still needed to verify and sign what was required so if I needed their services I had those arrangements made. I had our daughter Eden take me to the funeral home to finish up what requirements that were needed from me. I was able to get the urn that he had seen several years previous when he paid for his mothers' urn. He told me then, that is the urn I want when I die. I can't believe they still had it. But they did and that is the one we got for him just as he requested.

I did not want him embalmed. He had been poked and probed enough. I was going to have him cremated just as he and I had discussed. I also told the funeral director when he was cremated I wanted to be there. Michael was always there for others and I did not want him to be sent off alone. I knew he told me in his life until he met me there was never any family to show up to any event when he graduated anything, earned a medal, or if he was hurt and in the hospital. That was not the case during our life together. I was always there for him just as he was there for me. The next few days were rough waiting for the memorial. Our children were there every day with me, monitoring my state of mind, and just being supportive. I know they were concerned how I was going to react to losing him. They knew he was my whole world. They would tell me later they couldn't believe how well I handled it. Our friends would say the same thing. They didn't mean that I wasn't upset, it's just they didn't see me fall to pieces or worse. What they didn't know is that Michael had always told me I was the strongest person he has ever known. He told me no matter what I had to keep going, keep moving forward in life and that although I would be upset he knew I was strong. I keep reminding myself of that every time I get upset. Also most people don't see how absolutely heartbroken you are, the times you cry because you miss them when you are either in your car driving, in your room, or anytime by yourself. They don't see that, they see only what you let them see. Michael told me that I'm strong. I am strong, but I miss him horribly. I will miss him until the day I see him again.

I was anxious about the memorial. I didn't know how I would react. I didn't know if I would break down or hold it together. But the memorial was absolutely wonderful and emotional. I know he would have been proud. He used to tell me probably no one will show up to my funeral but it was a packed house. Most of our family which also included most of our grandchildren were there, Carlye, Daryn, Bryson, Kinsley, and McKayla were there. Our grandchildren that were toddlers, Kennedy, Christopher, Ellie and Rowan were not there as their parents thought they were too young. Our daughter Eden insisted on saying a few words at the memorial. She had worked diligently on it. She also read a poem. It was extremely emotional for her to do and I knew it had to be tough but it was also so loving, wonderful and moving for her to get up and share her feelings about the man who had been her dad for years. It brought tears to all in the room. Also many of the young adults whom he knew got up to say a few words about just how he had affected their life and how wonderful he was. Several were on the program to speak but others just felt compelled to get up and share stories of how wonderful Michael was and how he had impacted their life. Michael's brother, Paul, although emotional and broken-hearted I know, he also felt compelled to say a few words and share a story about him and Michael. It made us smile but also brought tears. Paul told of how Michael always told him to never kneel in life, stand tall, and he went on to tell that Michael had only knelt to one person in his life and that was his wife, Joyce. That really hit me hard because I knew how Michael was, I knew his philosophy and I knew he loved me with all his heart. Also one of the guys that stood up to say a few words was someone who had been around our family for years. In fact several of the guys that spoke, Jonathan and Casey had been around for years, they were friends with our son, Larry and we all looked at them as our family. They called us Mom and Dad. All the boys did. Another guy to speak as well, Connell was like the other boys who spoke, he was a friend to our son and our son had asked him to say a few words that Larry had sent Connell to say for him. Our son was unable to get up and neither could the rest of us as we were way too emotional. All the speakers were wonderful and heartfelt. It meant so much to me and our family and friends their touching words. It also would have made Michael really proud to see the love they had for him. It speaks volumes about the impact Michael had on others and the relationships he made and maintained. This is why so many showed up including people that most people wouldn't expect to see. Our ex son-in-law and his family whom we loved dearly, our much extended family which included in-laws of our children, Wayne and Jan who have been great friends to us throughout this journey. Wayne and Michael had been close since the 1980's. Rick, another friend Michael has known since the 1980's was there as well. Many other friends were there, many young people and of course our beloved church family that had been just wonderful to us were all there. And as an incredibly moving addition there were the patriot guard, the 21 gun salute, the presentation to me of the flag and a beautiful DVD tribute with some of his most favorite songs that played and at the same time showed some great photos of him throughout his life. It was a beautiful tribute and everyone in the room, young and old were all emotionally touched by the service and his life. After it was concluded many came up to hug me and give me their condolences. Several of his friends were telling me that they had so many great stories of Michael and had wished they could have shared them but they were just too emotional. One of Michael's friends, it seemed that he just had something important to tell me. He stood there in front of me for a long time and just couldn't find the words. Later he would call me to say that he had tried to find one bad memory or thing that Michael had ever done and he couldn't remember one. They were all funny, crazy or good. He told me it's hard to find someone like that. I agreed and was thankful he had shared that with me.

I went home after the service with several family members and waited for a few hours until it was time to meet the funeral director at the crematorium. I did not know what to expect, I just knew I had to be there. He deserved that. When the time came, our oldest daughter Christie, our oldest granddaughter Carlye, and our son Larry, met at the crematorium with the funeral director and the crematorium manager.

As the funeral director kept telling me you do not want to see him because the process of decay has probably started taking place. He went back and took several copies of Michael's fingerprint for us to have. I went back and forth in my mind about that but I still remembered how Michael went in with one of our sons' friends at his cremation and kissed him on the forehead before he was placed in the furnace. That was what made up my mind for me. I told the crematorium manager when he asked, Yes, I would like to see him. All of us decided we all wanted to see him. So we were escorted into a room where a particular type of gurney was with a long white cardboard box with a lid on top. And we all knew inside was Michael. As we stood beside the box the crematorium manager lifted the white top and there lying in a white linen wrapping with his head on a small white pillow was Michael. He had oil over his body. He looked so peaceful. Not anything like he looked at the hospital. His eyes were closed, mouth closed and he looked so very peaceful. I leaned down to kiss him on his forehead and told him I loved him and then the top of the box was placed back on the box and the box was lowered and placed into the furnace. The crematorium manager walked me over to a table to show me how the process is completed and how a tab and number will follow his remains forever now. I thanked the man and was grateful to be able to see him one last time.

I told the family that was there with me that he looked great. They all agreed they thought he looked great as well. And I was really glad that we came to send him off and especially glad we had them lift the top of the box so we could see how very peaceful he looked. I was told that I could pick him up the next day in his urn and I couldn't wait until I could pick him up and take him back home with me. I went home and called the rest of the family and told them how peaceful he looked and that I'm so glad I was able to see him one last time. I wish my brother could have been there because it had really upset him at the hospital to see after Michael died. I also wish our daughter Eden could have been there as well. It would have helped them emotionally to see him lying there peaceful.

The next day I picked him up and I must say it felt good knowing he was with me again. I had ordered a locket with his fingerprint on the front that I could wear with his remains inside with a transcription on the back that read "I Will Always Love You". Because we were waiting for the locket to come in the mail the funeral home did not glue the lid of the urn down but we taped it down until they could place some remains in the locket. After the locket came in then the urn was glued shut.

I also ordered all 3 of our children and 5 of our grandchildren a flat type medallion that also had his fingerprint on the front. On the back of each one was placed a transcription that was special to each of them, some were sayings that Michael would say to them, or something special to them to remember him by. These necklaces have been very special to us all. At times we have found ourselves holding the locket or medallion and thinking about him. It just gives us another level of comfort. It makes us feel he's near. I am so glad we had the funeral director get a copy of Michael's fingerprint so we could have these made.

Chapter Twenty One

The day after I picked him up was Christmas Eve. For our family this wasn't going to be the best Christmas but I knew I needed to try to be as cheerful as I could especially for my grandchildren. Our children went out of their way to try to make my day as good as it could be. We did laugh some; talked of some of Michael's funny jokes and we would all smile and think of him. But honestly there was a big hole in our family missing as anyone could guess. After we left my sons home where we all met for

Christmas Eve our oldest daughter and her family and I went to the Church that had been so good to us for Christmas Eve service and communion. It was a beautiful service and we were all glad we went. It was a beautiful church.

The next day I told my oldest daughter that we needed to all go to see the Christmas lights. We need to get out of the house. It had been an incredibly hard couple of years. It had been heartbreaking, emotional and I was battling pneumonia to top it off. But I knew that everyone in our house needed something positive so I told everyone "let's go see the Christmas lights." We decided to go and we were able to get some good pictures and we just really enjoyed seeing the lights. It put a smile on all of our faces. We also laughed at times and we all really needed that. After what we had experienced the last 21 months we knew more than anything life is short! Don't waste it!

In Closing, this journey I know had to happen for a reason. I believe that everything happens for a reason. God knows that mystery, I don't. But I do know that how Michael and I handled this journey together, and how I handle the journey after may have something to do with it. I don't know. I know it's hard to understand why Michael needed to leave this world. I will never understand that. I do know that I was lucky to have had the privilege of being Michael's wife for 23 years and his best friend for 29 years. I miss him and I believe I will always miss him. I also think it's important to speak his name, talk about the funny things he said and did, the movies he liked, how smart he was, and on and on. Michael did exist. Michael did make an impact in many peoples' lives. I remind my grandchildren things he would say about something we are doing and we will laugh. It makes us feel good and makes us feel that love we shared with him. You can talk about your loved one even if they are deceased, you can miss them and still love them. Just because someone dies doesn't mean you have to forget them. To some it's uncomfortable but I talk about Michael often, I have one of his voice mail messages as my ringtone so I can hear his voice as I have every day for 29 years. Everyone is different. I am aware of that. But I believe you have to do what makes you happy and what makes you comfortable. Whatever makes you feel better. Not what others think you need to do.

As far as his medical treatment I have questioned should we have kept doing the baking soda protocol through the whole treatment process, and I think probably we should have, except since his ph was 7, then I think it maybe would have put his ph too high unless we had just given him just a little bit. Then I wondered if his esophagus got punctured in the hospital the time before the last hospital stay. Also I question should we have taken the chemo treatments at all. Some people say you shouldn't. But in the end

I tell myself hindsight is 20/20. What I do know is comparing March 2014 when he was diagnosed and then Michael living to December 17, 2015, that is a miracle. We worked tirelessly to make that happen. We were able to spend 21 more months together. Many more than the doctors predicted. In the end Michael lost his life and I spent hours wondering how we could have extended it more. But all the pondering will not bring Michael back. I do appreciate many of the doctors and nurses that were so wonderful to us throughout this journey. They know who they are and they are all angels. Michael would tell them that.

I do hope this book helps anyone have an easier journey by finding some of the answers that we learned the hard way or just enforcing the fact that there is hope. New treatments come available every day. Do your research. Educate yourself. Don't give up. Miracles do happen all over the world every day.

Most importantly cherish every day because life is short and death comes for us all. Good luck and God Bless you all!

Chapter Twenty Two

This chapter is a listing of the items that we used throughout Michaels' cancer journey. I will post a general idea of how we used these in this chapter.

1) Bob Mills unrefined baking soda (found at health food stores)

2) Black Strap Molasses (found at health food stores)

3) Lugol's Iodine (found at health food stores)

4) Samento (online)

5) Frankincense topically (useful in some people for inflammation)

6) Pedialyte (While we were fighting this cancer other than the numerous challenges that we mentioned in the other chapters being able to go to the bathroom became a problem. Over several months he was prescribed lots of medicine to help with this problem. We had tried over the counter medicines but we always kept enemas on hand especially the ones with the extra fluid. His pain doctor even prescribed taking shots in his belly. Most of these options were hard on his system especially because his cancer was in his esophagus and the radiation was affecting his stomach as well. In the end what appeared to help him the most was Pedialyte. What was happening is he was dehydrated. Because he was taking tube feedings and they were mostly protein and because he was unable to consume enough water he would dry up internally. This created

challenge after challenge. Most of the time it stopped our effort to add more nutrition in his feeding tube. After months of trial and error the Pedialyte would hydrate his body and own his own he would be able to go to the bathroom. This is just a little tip in case you have similar challenges.

7) Benadryl – This medicine is good for side effects and nausea. It also is good for drying up secretions from allergies or sinus that can cause problems when your esophagus is closed.

8) Ginger Ale – This is really good for nausea. With all the medicine that you can use, Zofran that can be used under your tongue or liquid in a feeding tube or the medicine that is rubbed on your wrist, and benadryl, we added ginger ale which really helped stop the puking.

9) Ondestadron/Zofran – This is a nausea medicine that comes in a liquid form that can be put in a feeding tube or in a tablet that can be put under your tongue.

Chapter Twenty Three

Baking Soda, Black Strap, Iodine, Samento Protocol

Bob Mills purified baking soda at a health food store
Black strap molasses at a health food store
Nutramedix Samento Microbial Defense www.nutramedix.com

J Crow Lugol's Solution Iodine 2 %. www.jcrowmarketplace.com
or most health food stores
PH testing strips, we used brightcore nutrition. You can get these on
Amazon.
These testing strips have a range between 4.5 - 9.0

We would test his urine during the day, when he would get up, before he was taking any treatment, and an hour or so after treatment and at night. Also any time he went to the bathroom. The goal was to keep his ph up to 7.25-7.5 period. 7.5 ph was better than 7.25 ph. A 7.5 ph is where Cancer is kept dormant per the research I found. Every so often we would increase just enough baking soda and black strap molasses to reach a ph of 8.0-8.5 for 4 days. At 8.0 ph Cancer dies also per the research I found. Our goal was to never go over a ph of 8.5.

Depending on what the ph strips would show we would either make up 1/2 tsp or 1 tsp baking soda plus the same corresponding amount of black strap molasses with one cup of water warmed up for just long enough to feel warm. Michael would always take the protocol 2 hours before or after eating. To explain a little more in detail, if Michaels' pH was 5.5 or 6.0 we would give him 1 teaspoon of baking soda and 1 teaspoon of black strap warmed up in a cup of water on the stove just until the baking soda was dissolved. Then Michael would drink it down quick because he said it tasted terrible. Then he would put some truvia sweetener on his tongue to help him tolerate the taste. If his ph was 6.5 or 7.0 we would give him 1/2 of a teaspoon of baking soda and 1/2 of a teaspoon of black strap also warmed up in a cup of water on the stove. We would just play around with the amount we needed based on how much his ph would raise depending on how much he took. The goal was to keep him at 7.5 ph if at all possible.

Again, we did this protocol on and off for several months. We would just watch his ph on and off throughout the day. We would also every month or so raise his ph up to 8.0 and keep it there for 4-5 days multiple times. We did this by increasing just by a small amount the baking soda and black strap that Michael would take. We did not want to go over 8.5 ph. One time we did go over 8.5 ph and Michael said I do not feel good so we had him drink some apple juice to bring his ph down.

Although we didn't do this protocol every day, we would do maintenance if his ph would get low. After several months of this protocol his ph had been staying pretty steady at 7.5. Sometimes his ph would even be at an 8.0.

The first time he had taken the baking soda protocol and when we got his ph up to 8.0 and kept it for 4 days, the fourth day was a little rough on him. Michael felt out of it. Noises would come out of his esophagus. The theory is that 7.5 pH keeps Cancer dormant. A 8.0 ph kills Cancer cells and when they die they let off carbon dioxide. This is where the term "kill the cancer and not the patient" comes from. We had to monitor him close to make sure we didn't need to give him some apple juice or even take him to the doctor. But he would be fine.

Also during this time Michael took 1 dropper of lugol iodine with 15 drops of Samento every day. We put the iodine and the Samento with b12 into cranberry grape juice or the equivalent. Not much, just a small amount of the juice. Michael would take this almost every day all throughout the 21 months even if we had to pour it into his feeding tube. Once in a while he would take a week off here and there. But he insisted on taking this as well. He called it his Trojan horse against Cancer.

I made sure to keep away from microwaving any food or drink. We used Stevia or a Truvia sweetener. We watched and monitored what the foods he ate based on what would lower his ph. There was a chart online that showed what type of foods were in what pH group. It was pretty interesting to see and it reinforced the reason people that could actually eat were eating a lot of salads and other foods that were in a high alkaline diet to keep their pH up. These were the people that were having the best results beating cancer or a better chance of putting cancer into remission.

The goal for us moving forward was to keep his pH at a 7.25-7.5 level. 7.5 pH was always the best. We would reach a time with the iodine and Samento that every time we checked his pH he would be steadily in the 7's. His oxygen level would also be in the 98 or 99%. This was where we wanted to keep him. We monitored his oxygen with a little gadget we got from a pharmacy that went on his finger.

Keeping tabs on his ph was critical. Cancer thrives in low oxygen and low pH level. These items that we were using would help create an environment that Cancer does not like or does not thrive in.

Everyone is different. We had to play around to see how each different type dose would affect Michaels' pH levels. We got pretty confident in what amount he needed and became able to keep his pH up to the levels we needed to maintain.

** Again, I am not a doctor and I am not suggesting to anyone that they try what we had used. I am just sharing what protocol Michael was using to beat Cancer. Although he didn't beat Cancer entirely we do believe it bought him many more months of life. I know there are studies out there right now at several Cancer research centers to see the effect that baking soda has on cancer. I hope and pray that a cure for all types of Cancers will be found and that no person or family will have to ever endure the pain and heartbreak of Cancer.

Chapter Twenty Four

The following pictures are as follows left to right.

1)   Thanksgiving 2010 with Mark (Joyce's brother), Big Mo (Joyce's Dad), and Michael (proud as can be) This picture so how very big Michael was.

2)   Michael and Joyce dancing 2012

3)   Michael & Joyce at Easter 2014

4)   Dad, Michael, Joyce and Mom at the Proton Therapy Center

5)   Michael & Joyce (Michael ringing the bell Graduating Proton Therapy

6)   Michael & Joyce at Proton Graduation Lunch with Doctors and staff. Michael wanted to thank the doctors and staff for all their help and care.

7)   Michael & Joyce driving to get the port placed for 2nd Chemo round

8)   Michael and Joyce at the end of 2015 when he was very weak

9)   Michael when he got his wings on 12/17/2015

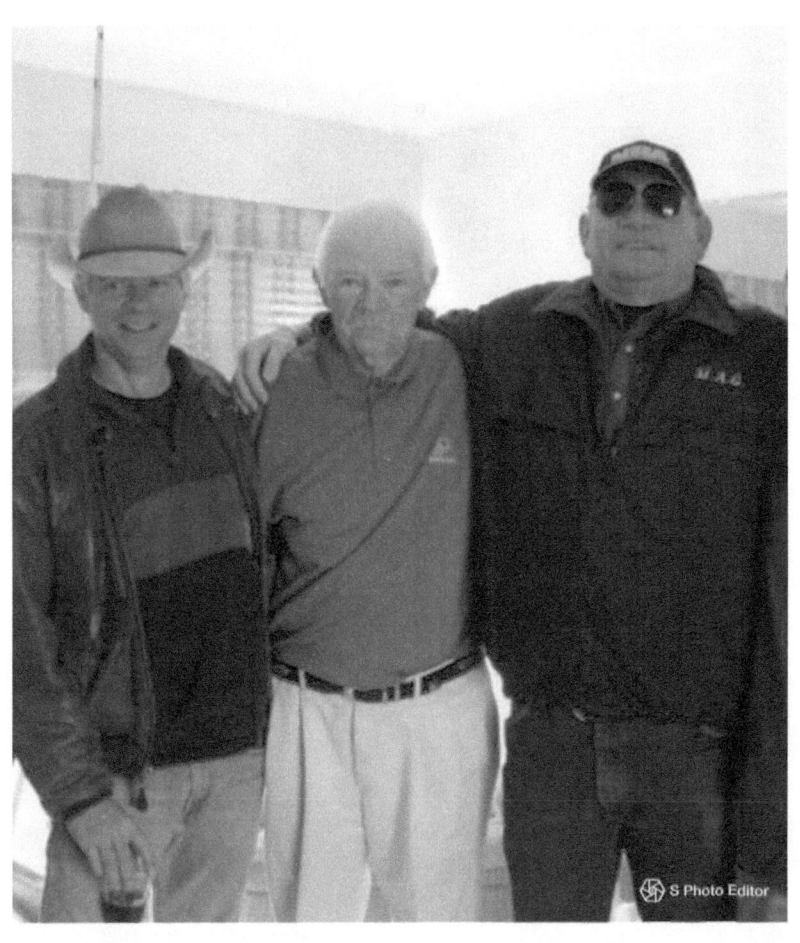

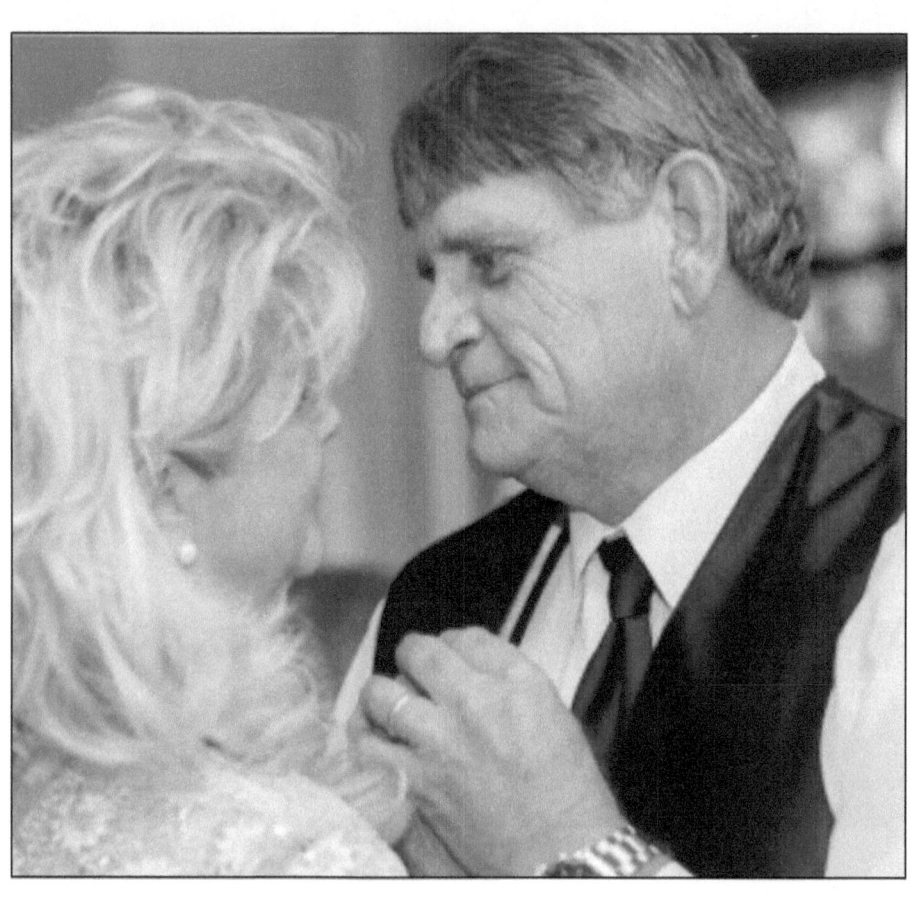

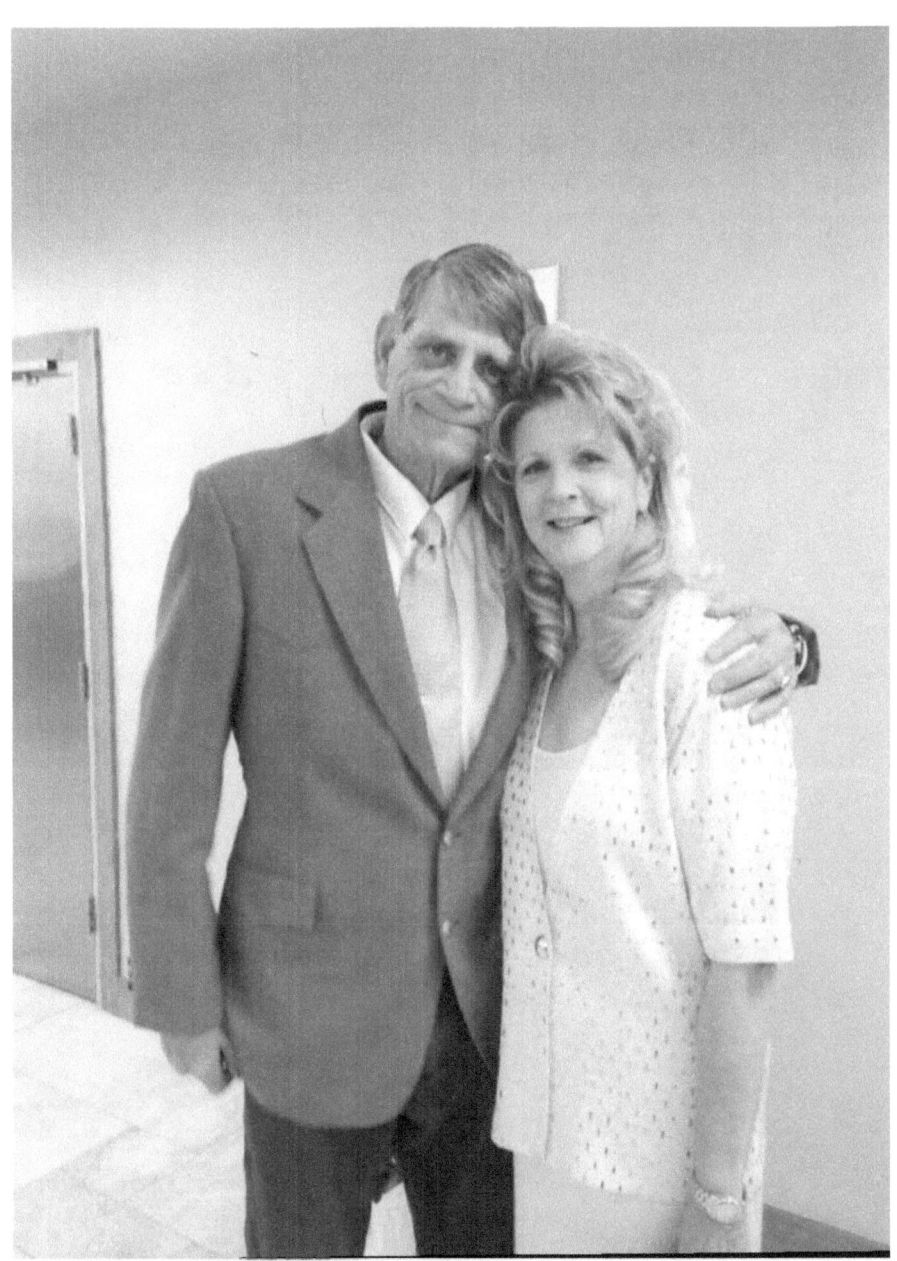

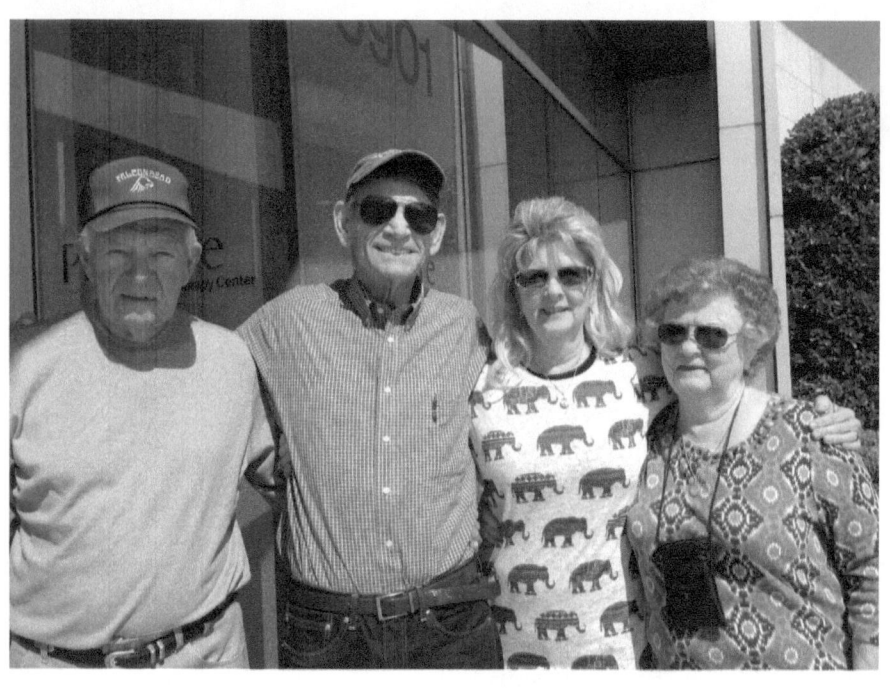

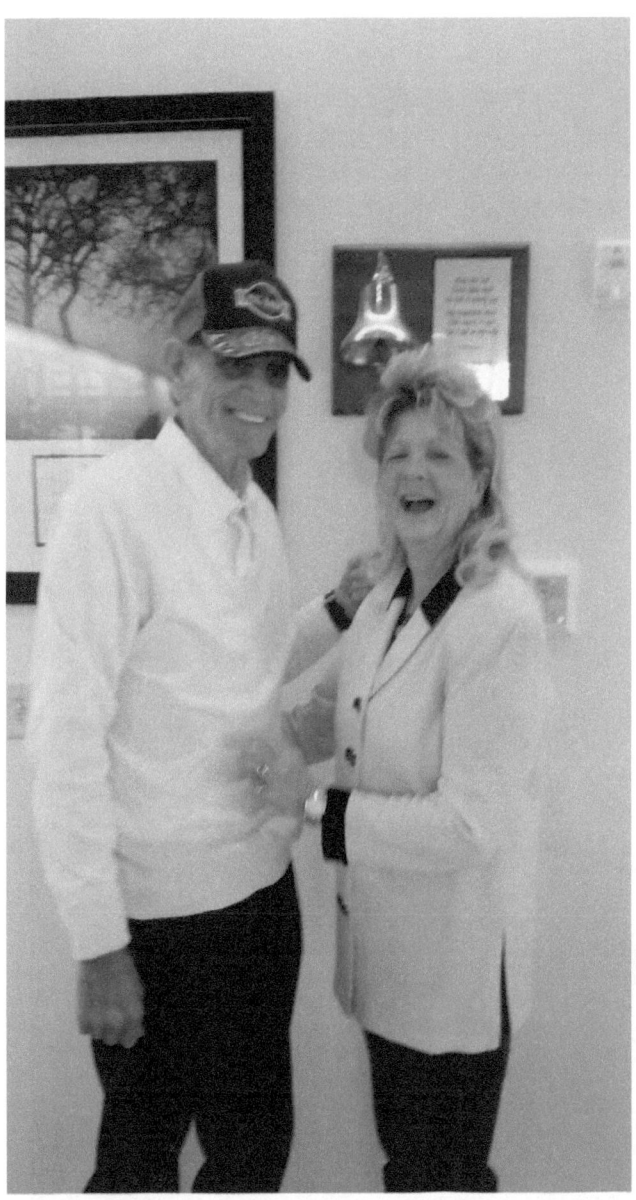

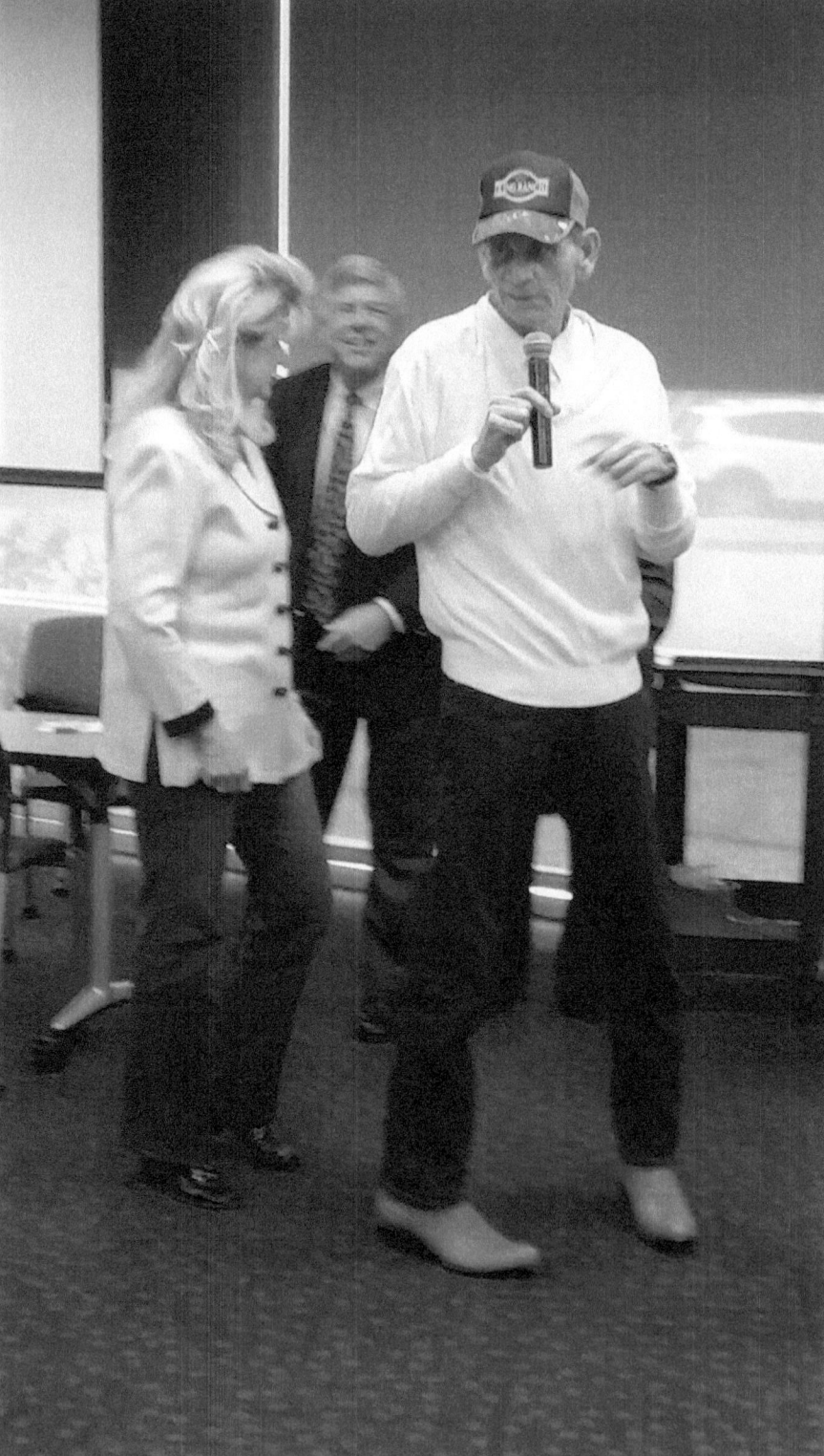

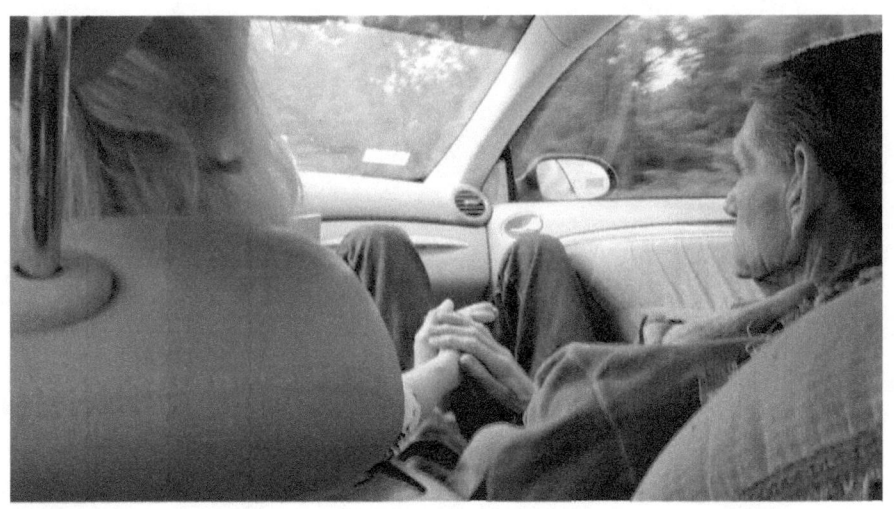

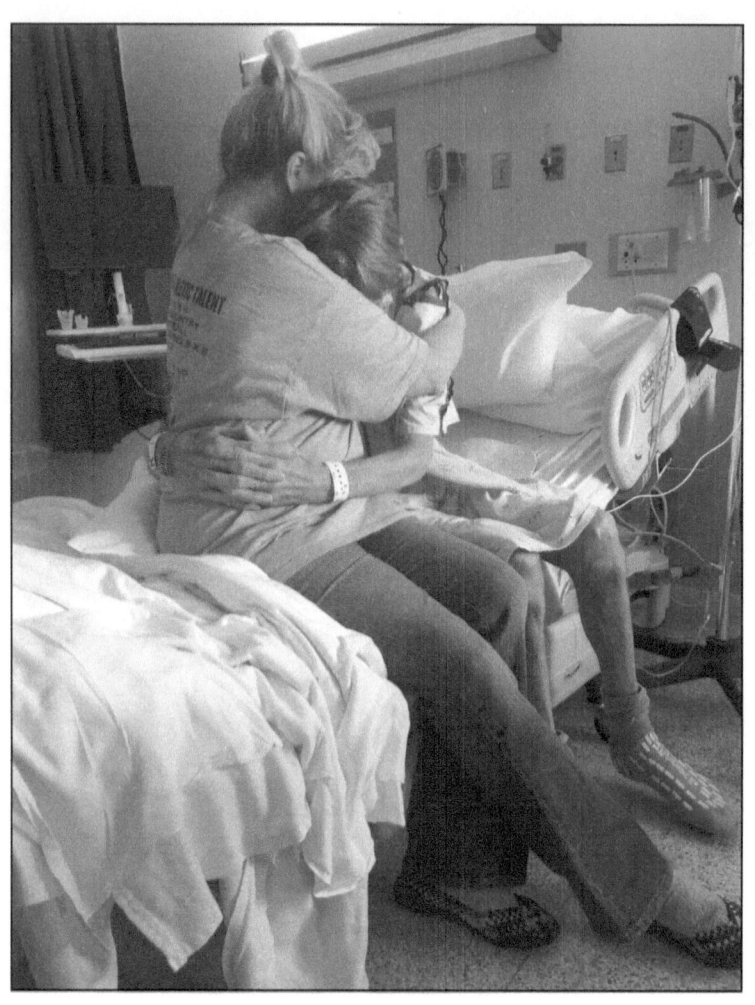

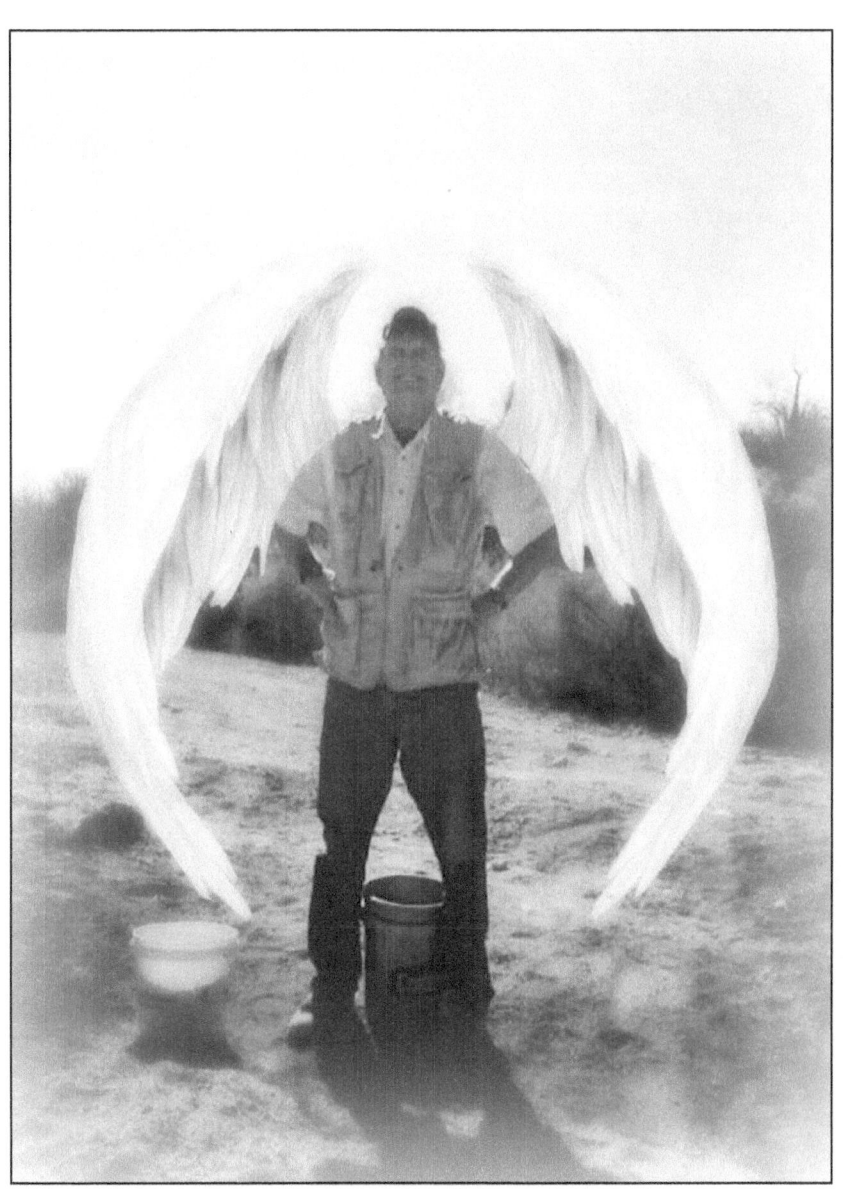